FOR PEETE'S SAKE

The Biography of
Calvin Peete
Champion Golfer

written by
Dolly Ness

For Peete's Sake: The Biography of Calvin Peete, Champion Golfer

Copyright © 2008 by Dolly Ness

All rights reserved. Printed in the United States of America. This book may not be reproduced in any manner (electronically or hard copy) without written permission from the author.

Write to Dolly Ness, 209 SE 35th St., South Beach, OR 97366 for more information.

ISBN: 978-1-893471-19-1

Library of Congress Control Number: 2008938033

1. Biography   2. Golf   3. Sports Heroes

Published in the United States by Rushford and Associates Denver, CO.

Cover design by Deborah Gotto

Photos provided by Calvin Peete and Dolly Ness

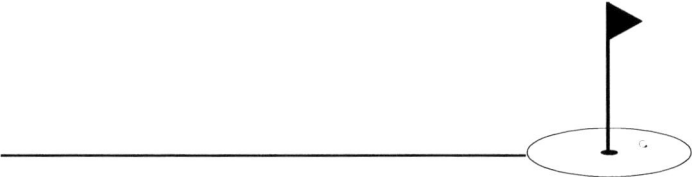

Acknowledgments

Friends play an important part in almost everyone's life. They play a huge part in mine. This book owes its life to my dear friend Carrolle Rushford, who is also a friend to Calvin and Pepper. We owe her our debt of gratitude for placing her trust and confidence in Calvin's story of worth and my ability to tell it.

My dear friend, and often mentor, Frances Caldwell, edited and formatted and encouraged me along the way to the end of this book. Ed Corcoran also played a huge role in editing.

Of course I'm indebted to Calvin who shared his life's story with me, and his wife Pepper who kept him on track and corresponded with answers to all my questions.

Most important is my husband, Troy Ness. Without his unflinching support and certainty in my ability to see this to the end I would have given up long before I began.

To my mother,

not a day goes by . . .

A Message From Calvin

Hi, this is Calvin Peete. I started my life from very humble beginnings being one of 19 children by my father's two marriages. I was the one who was most unlikely to succeed.

Although I have been through many trials and tribulations which you will read about in this book, they did not stop me from becoming successful. With hard work, determination, perseverance and knowing your life has purpose no matter your current circumstances you can win at the game of life just as I did.

I hope you enjoy my life's journey.

Calvin Peete

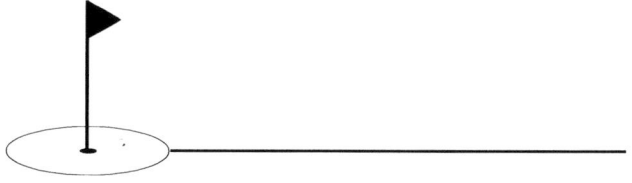

In the Beginning

Detroit was the fourth-largest city in the nation in the 1930s, largely due to the automotive industry. In the 1940s it had become part of the war machine as WWII forced the automakers to re-tool and prepare tanks and equipment for battles. The country was losing the war but Detroit had geared up; things were about to change, and not just in the battlefields across the ocean.

General Motors employed 450,000 people, up from 303,000. Ford grew to 200,000, including an unprecedented 25,000 women among the 100,000 employees of its bomber plant. In the same era Chrysler increased its employees to 130,000 compared to its previous high of 65,000. News stories described production lines miles long. Chrysler was making at least $675,000,000 worth of tanks, planes and guns in 1942. Ford had eleven miles of airplane runways at Willow Run heightening all efforts to make America's war machine the biggest, the best, the fastest. America, and especially Detroit, was a fine tuned machine.

However, not everything was good in Detroit. In the spring of 1943, three Black workers at a Detroit Packard auto plant, which had been retrofitted to manufacture aircraft engines, were promoted to the formerly all-white job of metal polisher. Up until that time, Black workers in the Detroit auto plants were kept in the most low-paying, dirty, and dangerous jobs–often in the ferociously hot foundries. White workers, 20,000 of them, went on a week–long racist strike known as the "Packard hate strike."

That June, race fights between Blacks and whites broke out at Belle Isle, Detroit's largest integrated recreation park. Over the next 36 hours, 34 people were killed and 25 of them Black, and at least 17 of the Blacks were killed by police because they sided with the white mobs. Hundreds more were injured or jailed.

A young Black man, Charlie Sifford, was drafted into the Army in 1943 and sent to Okinawa after his basic training. He survived the war and before being discharged formed a golf team. Golf, a sport for rich white men, was now being noticed and played by non-rich Blacks, largely through the effort of Charlie Sifford. Charlie fought the race issue constantly as a Black golfer, an amazing Black golfer. It would be his cross to bear that he would be turned away constantly from playing major tournaments because he was Black. He left the South in order to get at least some of the recognition he deserved. He was to be a trailblazer for a young Black boy, Calvin Peete, born July 18, 1943, in Detroit to Dennis Peete, an automobile factory worker, and Irenia Bridgeford Peete, a housekeeper. Black, by the way, is the term preferred by Calvin, rather than African American and so will be used for his biography.

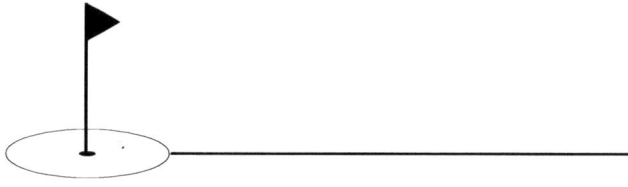

Calvin's Childhood

Detroit life for young Calvin was good, or at least good in comparison to much of the rest of his young life. The country shifted gears again and the economy continued to grow. However, the nation's prosperity didn't trickle down to the poorer segments of society, including Calvin's family. Even so he still looks back on most of this time as the best moments of his life. In this he is fortunate as many young Black children from this era can't recall pleasant times during the impoverishment that racism afflicted upon them. His demeanor brightens as he retells the fun times in Detroit.

The only drawback Calvin saw at this childhood time was going to school–never a priority for him, a deficiency he regrets, and a paradox in his retelling. The school memories he does relate are generally unhappy, and he prefers instead to recall the happier times with friends and family.

The vacant lot across from his east side Detroit home, the "bumble bee lot" as the kids knew it, was a big summer attraction for catching bumble bees. They caught them in mason jars and kept them, but as he laughingly recalls, "I don't even know why we kept them. We sure didn't eat them or play with them 'cuz we would get stung. But it sure was fun!" Making their own games and amusements kept Calvin and the neighborhood kids busy. There were no camps; organizations were usually for the richer kids, and poor Black children relied on their own resources for diversions.

Playing mumbly-peg was another great sport–flipping a knife or ice pick off your finger tip or other body part so that it would stick in a designated spot. Marbles was another favorite game of Calvin's, probably because he was good at it. Maybe the games that required eye-hand coordination was a sign that Calvin would be as focused and competitive in these types of sports later in life.

Winters found him and his brothers looking for stray dogs to bring home to the barn in back of their house where they would hook them up like Huskies to pull their sleds. The end of that came when chasing a small dog he slipped and fell on a piece of glass, ripping open his left hand resulting in stitches. That wasn't the worst that would happen to Calvin in a lifetime of tribulations.

Perhaps as a result of his lack of interest in school, he was eventually talked into playing hooky and introduced to the "seedier" side of life. He joined other kids from the neighborhood to steal from markets and warehouses and sell the products on the street. Joe, a friend of his brother, had an unhealthy influence on Calvin, and once talked him into distracting sales people while Joe stole a rifle by sticking it down his pants leg. Calvin admits to being scared to death and vowed never to do it again, even though they reaped a cash reward at the early age of eight or nine. Calvin's parents were aware that Joe was not a boy to be trusted and when Calvin continued to hang around with him and was found out by his mother, he received the worst whipping of his childhood. It did not, however, deter him from making more wrong choices in his youth.

Colorful lives crop into Calvin's childhood memories. Butch and Spider, cousins and thieves, frequently stole from Calvin. One day he decided he'd had enough. He jumped them and beat them up as they came past his house on their way to school and that was the end of that! Calvin remembers this as being fair, making them "atone for their sins." As J.C. Penney once said, "I would never have amounted to anything were it not for adversity. I was forced to come up the hard way." Calvin was forced to come up the hard way, too.

Although some of his memories include pastimes that were not always above the law, and certainly beyond what would be expected for a child's play, Calvin remembers that early neighborhood and house fondly. Catching bees and butterflies, playing marbles and jumping rope were all normal signs that Calvin's earlier childhood was good. He also admits to doing all the "normal" stuff young boys sometimes do— childhood pranks like breaking a few windows and stealing from a few gardens.

He had neighborhood buddies and a stable family; they had friends who came by and stayed for dinner. There was a sense of harmony and protection that would take most of his life to find again. There was food on the table; a phone that was never disconnected; a neighbor's TV to watch "Frankenstein," "Dracula," "The Lone Ranger," and other shows;

clothes on their backs which were seldom new; and they were happy. He and his siblings were each other's best friends and Calvin never saw a need to form any other close attachments. It was also a time in life when church wasn't an option; it was a priority. He could occasionally skip school or make other excuses for not being where he was expected, but there was no excuse for missing church. Both his mother and father were religious and had church meetings at their house, introducing the teachings of Jesus to the children at an early age.

The family always had pets and one dog especially was a strong protector of his mother. That little dog would sit under Calvin's mama's chair and growl and glare at anyone who approached, including the children. A cat they had was a good mouser, but unfortunately it brought the mice home alive to play with for a while before doing away with them. Calvin remembers napping with her as a child until one day she disappeared. Then he brought home a stray dog, a cocker spaniel. Calvin recalls that Trixie was a fun dog who gave him many hours of enjoyment as well as the responsibility of feeding and cleaning up after his dog's messes. Unfortunately, Trixie also liked to chase cars until one winter when a car couldn't stop on the ice and ran over her. Memories of Calvin's first dog bring back a look of loss to his eyes, maybe of those happy childhood days, as well as the dog.

The house they lived in wasn't large but was adequate and comfortable even though the six children all shared beds. When cousins or friends came to visit they slept on pallets or the floor. Calvin never realized until he was grown that in reality they were living in poverty. His father established the ground rules, and bickering among the siblings wasn't allowed–they were family and family stuck together. If there was a disagreement with brothers and sisters they were expected to settle it among themselves and not involve their father, or even let him hear of it. "Don't mess with the Peetes" was the rule in the neighborhood, too, because if someone messed with one Peete, they had the rest of them to deal with.

Another house rule was to respect their elders. Every mother in his neighborhood was like his mother, every father like his father. "Yes sir," was how elders were addressed even on the east side, tough side of Detroit. These early lessons in conduct contributed to Calvin's demeanor in his later years on the golf course as he was often referred to as a gentleman on the golf course.

Calvin was closest to his brother Aaron at that time, Calvin being the youngest and Aaron two years older. They both wanted to have money, but Aaron was the industrious one who always found work, employing his other brothers and sisters from time to time. Dennis was the oldest of the sons, and he watched out for his siblings, even cautioning Calvin against smoking, a warning Calvin wished he'd heeded. Of course, it was expected that the older siblings take care of the younger ones, and at that time Calvin was the youngest. He readily admits that he was happy to take advantage of that position whenever he could, seeking his mother whenever an opportunity for revenge against a sister or brother who didn't give in to him.

One afternoon, his sister Irene was left in charge of Calvin when his parents were out. While he napped she went next door to visit friends. Of course she knew better, but she was a typical child and thought she knew it all. When Calvin awoke and found himself alone in a darkening house he became frightened. His parents came home to see a crying child, unattended, and the ending was written. When Irene came home she received the punishment due the crime—a spanking. Naturally he was never again left alone again by his siblings.

Both of Calvin's parents worked hard to support their large family. Neither was educated but they always found jobs and had good work ethics. Calvin's mother worked in a canning factory for a while but most of the time worked as a domestic who cleaned houses for wealthier families. When she had to work on weekends and the employer's family had children, Calvin was allowed to go with her to play with the other children; this ultimately had an influence on his outlook on life. He knew there were those who lived in a life style very unlike his and the idea began to germinate that he would like to live more like those people. His father worked in the factories. One factory, Dodge-Maine, had family day once a year, when families could see the factory assembly line. Calvin also had some comparisons then of what the haves and have-nots tasted of life. His parents never took real vacations, choosing instead to work so that school clothes could be provided for their burgeoning family. Calvin was realizing that he wanted more out of life and that this was going to be a difficult goal to achieve given his present living situation.

Eventually the family moved to the west side of Detroit, just off 14th Street, amid an undercurrent of marital turmoil. Even though the neighborhood was better, Calvin found that friends were hard to find there. Unfortunately, soon after their move, his mother and father separated, his father leaving the family behind. In spite of this, Calvin feels that he had a caring family and that both his mother and father were involved and loving parents.

However, the only really good thing Calvin remembers about this now more difficult time was that he met the famous boxer, Joe Louis. When Calvin was about nine he and his brother were coming home from the library when they saw Louis at the market. They lined up much like groupies do today in freezing Detroit weather to meet him. He looked like a giant to little Calvin. He'd like to be like Joe Louis one day, not a fighter he thought, but famous and really good at something, and, of course, that surely would also bring fame and fortune. Little did young Calvin know that the golf bug had bitten Joe Louis hard, some say to the detriment of his boxing career. How that chance meeting and hopeful thought is the amazing story of Calvin Peete's life. His fame would become a reality and how much Joe Louis would again be linked to his life remains impressive to this day.

When Calvin's father left the family his mother had a hard time coping. Nobody talked about why his father left but Calvin was old enough to know that his questions would not be met with answers. He had no worries about what was going to happen to him; his young mind filled only with the thoughts of a loved child. "Daddy's not coming home" was enough to satisfy his curiosity. His mother and father never revealed why they separated but his mother told him, "Don't hold nothing against your daddy, he's a good man," and Calvin never did.

When he was a grown man Calvin did ask his father why he had left them. The reply was, "I left Detroit because I didn't want to kill Dennis." As the oldest son, Dennis had felt that he was responsible for mediating any arguments between his parents, assuming that he should step up he ultimately wanted to fight his father. At one point it was so bad the police were called, when Dennis was about sixteen. It just was almost more than Calvin's father could do to keep a strong and husky Dennis down. However, the fact that his father left the home didn't cure the need Dennis had for violence. Eventually he was shot dead in a pool room brawl after a continuing history of violent behavior.

In their new single-parent environment Calvin's sisters Irene and Margaret, still only a baby, along with Calvin, were still young enough to need adult supervision. His older siblings were basically in charge of taking care of themselves. Aaron went to live with a relative of his father's. Dennis came to the house every night, but the family was disrupted and there was a general mood of disquiet. At the time they lived in a house on Butternut Street that had a coal furnace with a coal feeder. Calvin recalls one winter night in that house the coal didn't burn, releasing carbon monoxide fumes into the house. Those in the house were saved by a neighbor who smelled what Calvin recalls as fumes, but what was probably smoke from the simmering coal. The fire department was called, and Calvin and his siblings were rescued from certain death. Surely that neighbor must have been proud then for saving this unfortunate family. Who knows, he also may have realized later that he had saved the life of a true champion.

By the following summer Calvin's mother wasn't able to work enough to support the family. Living on welfare caused her such severe depression that she also wasn't able to pay attention to the family that needed her. When she sent Calvin to register in school he played hooky for several weeks before his mother discovered his absence. Calvin was pretty good at avoiding things he didn't want to do and he really didn't want to go to school. To make sure that he got to school his mother had his sister Irene take him to enroll. It wasn't much use though as he only attended that school for about a month before they moved again.

This time they went to Calvin's uncle's house in Benton Harbor, Michigan, what was then a small, mostly Black community on the shores of Lake Michigan. This, too, proved to be only temporary and Calvin's life was to be disrupted once again, with severe consequences. Within a couple of weeks the uncle gave them money for bus tickets to Hayti, Missouri, to stay with their maternal grandmother, the only grandparent Calvin ever knew.

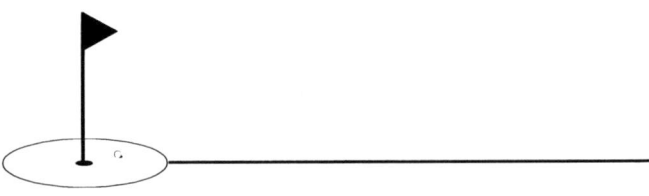

The Really Hard Times

Thus began Calvin's real culture shock, his horror, coming from the large metropolitan areas to live in the rural country. Even though they had visited there before, when eleven-year-old Calvin, year-old Margaret, and sixteen-year old Irene, (and necessary baby sitter) moved to the South he was in for a rude awakening. His other older brothers and sisters stayed in Detroit as they were considered old enough to take care of themselves. Perhaps they knew that living with their grandmother was not in their best interests, or maybe they were just lucky.

Hayti was definitely NOT Detroit. No more electric lights or indoor plumbing, a true loss of all the amenities Calvin was used to, even as a poor boy from Detroit. No sidewalks or paved streets, only outhouses, candle light, leaky roofs—a far cry from the luxuries of suburban life. Calvin was finally old enough to realize that the cotton that he was now required to pick wasn't manufactured, that it grew in the fields, and he had to work hard pulling it from the sticky plants. The only chickens he had seen in Detroit had been fried and now he was required to feed live ones. He saw his first mules plowing the fields, and drank milk that came straight from cows, not cold and pasteurized in bottles straight from the store.

Calvin remembers his first day in his new school as being horribly embarrassing and humiliating. He enrolled late, this time not because he was playing hooky, but because he was working in the cotton fields a little longer so that he had enough money to buy school clothes and shoes. In front of the other students his teacher asked him why he was so late enrolling, and when he replied honestly, they smirked and giggled at his poverty. Calvin's pain at those memories shows clearly on his face, a man now full of pride at his accomplishments, but ever mindful of the price of poverty on his young life.

When Calvin was still only eleven, his Aunt Lula took mercy on him and had him join her on a migrant trip. They worked in Suttons Bay, Michigan, to pick cherries when cotton picking was over in the South. This was perhaps a defining stop in the journey that would lead to Calvin's ultimate success. A cherry tree limb that Calvin was perched on suddenly broke and he fell. He landed on his left elbow, breaking it in three places. Calvin was rushed to the doctor in excruciating pain where the doctor in Michigan did an amazing job of putting Calvin's arm back together. However, his cherry picking was limited by the now ever-present cast.

When they returned to Missouri, Calvin went to the doctor to have the cast removed. The doctor drew them a diagram of how the arm had been broken, and even he was surprised that the Michigan doctor had been able to pin the fractures together so successfully. The only problem that soon became apparent was Calvin's inability to fully extend or fully bend his left elbow. This seemed like a small price to pay considering that an alternative would have been for him to have had his arm amputated. There were those people later in his life who would call this handicap a blessing in disguise. However, Calvin assures us he has never cared to eat cherries again.

Nonetheless, once back in Missouri Calvin got no special treatment because of his slight handicap. Even though he had lots of cousins and aunts living close by, Calvin's arrival as the oldest grandson heralded his era of being a male Cinderella. He was the one that was called on to chop wood, bring in coal, make the fires, and pump water. He eventually learned how to do all these to their expectations, but only after hearing all their hollering when he did them wrong.

Kind words seemed not in the vocabulary of his aunts and grandmother, at least none were offered to Calvin. To add to the humiliation he was required to pick out the switch to get whipped when he didn't do something quite right or in the expected time frame. At this point we could say we know life was hard but lots of boys had a hard life. But not all boys had the odds continue to mount and still survive to beat them in such an outstanding display of skill and perseverance.

Not long after Calvin's mother, Irenia, moved with Calvin and his sisters to Missouri, she left the children behind and moved to Chicago to find work, living with one of her sisters. When that failed to work out, she returned to Missouri, reclaimed her children, and found a small home down the block from Calvin's grandmother. Their existence was meager at best. While life was horrid when his mother was gone, it improved little with her return. Sometimes Calvin was sent to his grandmother's for food for his sisters and him.

One time he heard one of his aunts remarking that Irenia, his now poverty-stricken mother, should get a man so the children didn't have to come get food from them. This hurt Calvin so deeply that he skipped school frequently, once again playing hooky but now so that he could earn money. He would strip copper wire from burned-out huts and sell it for 22 cents a pound or pick pecans where he could get 33 cents a pound.

He recalls one day when he spotted a loaded pecan tree once on his way to school and decided to play hooky to pick those pecans. Try as he might he found he couldn't reach the first branch to climb it. So he walked to a nearby store that was frequented by winos and persuaded one of them to help him. Back at the pecan tree the man boosted him up and collected the pecans that Calvin dropped and shook from the tree. (No, he didn't fall from the tree again.) They spent most of that day picking pecans. They made about $34 for their hard work of picking almost a hundred pounds of pecans which they split evenly. When Calvin gave the money, a small fortune to their poverty-stricken family, to his mother she thanked him but reminded him that what she really wanted him to do was to go to school.

They weren't settled in Hayti long before Calvin's mother left once again, this time going back to Detroit. And once again Calvin was left with his grandmother, but now he was living in the small leaky shack behind her house. Constantly on his mind was how he was going to escape from what he refers to as a "hell hole." He spent as much time as he could with his mother's brother, Uncle Fred, who was a frequent patron of bars and gambling halls. Calvin usually got whipped for this alliance with Fred because his grandmother considered Fred a bad influence. Then Fred moved back with the family displacing Calvin from the shack, moving him from bad to worse, a porch of his aunt's two-bedroom shack. At night he froze on the couch he slept on, as the heat was only for his aunt's family in the house. He could see stars through the slats on the roof, and when it rained he had trouble finding a dry spot on the couch. Life for this young boy was miserable.

The last straw was when hungry Calvin helped himself to some peanut butter on the counter. His aunt discovered his breach and whipped him severely, punishment for allowing himself to act as a human being. At that he knew he had to escape. He ran away.

The first night on his own he slept in a car not knowing what he would do next. Then he remembered his Aunt Lula, the one who had taken him cherry picking, his father's sister, lived nearby and he went to her. She welcomed him with open arms, kept him warm and dry and safe and loved. He doesn't remember how long he was with Lula but some time later his father came to get him. Calvin is sure the church deacon wrote his father to come save the boy. His father arrived at another sister's house, sent for Calvin, and his rescue from the torture of his grandmother and the poverty of Hayti was finally over.

Life with Father

Despite his enormous relief that he no longer had to live with his grandmother he cried because they couldn't take his sister Margaret. So at age fourteen Calvin moved with his father to Pahokee, Florida, and a new life. There he joined his father's second family of three children, Alvin, another son named Dennis and Almeta, all younger than him. His stepmother, Ceatris, who had left three children from a previous marriage, had seven more during her marriage to Dennis, Calvin's father. In all Calvin's father had eighteen children.

Later in his life, Calvin's mother explained that she had left her youngest children because she had hoped to make a good enough living to be able to support them. She even wrote to Calvin, but her letters were never received, at least not by Calvin. He saw her about six years later when he was working in Detroit for a few weeks. At that time she was living with Calvin's brother and was suffering from poor health. She died in 1978 of a heart attack when she was living with her daughter Irene.

"When I moved to my father's, I was in the fifth or sixth grade and I wasn't interested in school." Moving from Detroit, then Missouri, and then to Pahokee, south Florida, was more than just many physical moves, they were educational moves—backwards. In Missouri he experienced harsh treatment for slight mistakes. Even a misspelled word could bring a beating with a fan belt from a car's engine. It's not difficult to see why Calvin skipped school often and ultimately didn't finish his formal education. He had little to no encouragement and few reasons to be in attendance.

In one history class Calvin drew an outline of the United States and the assignment was to fill in the states. He made his young artist's rendition of that map and penciled his name at the top. He then missed a few days of school, and on returning he looked for his map which the class was still working on. He looked around the room and finally found it in the possession of a cute little classmate. When he looked carefully at the map he saw his name had been erased and her name substituted. He accused her of taking it and demanded its return. Hearing the ruckus, the teacher asked what the problem was and when Calvin told the teacher that the girl had his map, the response was "Get out of my class." Calvin saw that girl many years later at a tournament and they spoke but never mentioned the incident. She probably didn't even remember it and Calvin was too much a gentleman to remind her. However, it is obvious that this incident still brings memories of the magnitude of inequitable treatment he suffered throughout his life, and that even the respect and fame he has achieved cannot completely erase all the bad times.

In Pahokee's Eastgate Middle School, Calvin was repeating subject matter he'd already learned in third and fourth grades. He felt that the teachers were not interested in teaching, only in getting their salaries. "You dress like you're the principal or something" was the attitude that the teachers had when Calvin arrived in his Florida school dressed in the manner of Detroit, with dress pants and shirt, Stacy Adams-like shoes. Never one to let other's perceptions of him color his ability to speak out Calvin once was ejected from class for voicing his understanding of the pronunciation of Ponce de Leon, which he learned as a French pronunciation in Detroit, and a far cry from the Southern dialect.

Repeatedly in school Calvin was reprimanded for speaking up and voicing his objections and opinions over what was being taught. Frustrated and discouraged it is not surprising that he chose to attend less and less. Finally in the eighth grade he realized that he was not going to pass mainly because of his poor attendance.

Still harboring his young boy's dream of one day going to law school, he knew he had to graduate. Somewhere along the way, he failed to understand that attendance was a requirement for that. So he had to take matters into his own hands. He took the initiative to schedule a meeting with Principal Morrell to address the situation. In the meeting he asked the unprecedented...to be allowed to join his classmates as they moved to the next grade level. He promised if he could not keep up he could be demoted to taking the eighth grade again. Of course, that didn't fly.

Mr. Morrell explained to Calvin that such a move simply would not be fair to the rest of the students who had been attending regularly. Repeated arguments from Calvin were of no avail. "Request denied," is the painful retort that Calvin remembers. At that point he told him, "Mr. Morrell, I won't be back to school." Calvin got up and walked out. Even though he quit school at that point, and that refusal of opportunity continues to be the greatest disappointment of his childhood, he has remained committed to acquiring knowledge and skills through study and experience throughout his life.

When Calvin wasn't attending school, most often playing hooky, he was walking the streets, usually alone or in the pool halls or craps houses, somewhere gambling. That was his life at fifteen. A dropout with only an eighth grade education, he started using the skills he had learned to gamble and play pool to help his father support his family. He became a good pool hustler, not great—we're not talking Minnesota Fats here, but good.

Eventually he even managed a pool hall in Pahokee, known as Big Henry's or "The Jitterbug" pool room where mostly young people hung out. This could have been where Calvin's story ends but as he says, "I looked at this situation the same as I looked at picking in the cotton, potato, and corn fields. I did not see myself or my future there."

Even though Calvin moved on from the pool halls, it should be remembered that pool is a skill that requires calculating angles and vectors to make the successful shots. It could be that the training and experience he gained from pool was the groundwork for his success in knowing where the ball trajectory would travel and spin.

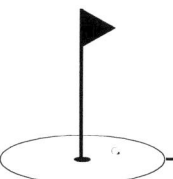

The Restless Years

Calvin feels that at that point he learned a valuable life lesson, but not the one the average person would take from such disappointment. The people who a young boy should be able to expect to be role models didn't fulfill that role, and the life he had lived was no cause for hope. What he did learn was that he should expect no favors or special treatment no matter what the circumstances. His take on life was that it was up to him to work as hard as he could to be the best that he could be. Those were very trying times, but he accepted that life would somehow work itself out. He applied for a job as a golf caddie, not knowing anything about golf, but was turned down. He picked corn with his father to help support the family but eventually turned to the gambling life.

Now we're not talking about the type of gambling that the average person goes to a casino for, but professional gambling, and not always aboveboard. When the dice were thrown, Calvin knew what they were going to be. He wasn't just shuffling and dealing the cards—he knew what everybody had. That's a professional gambler and hustler, and he was good. When Calvin decides to do something he does it well and with gusto.

People sought him out to partner with him. Otis Jones and Nathaniel Johnson, nicknamed Stitch, were his partners when he was sixteen and seventeen years old. They hung out together, played basketball together, even went to the same school before Calvin dropped out, and learned the same tricks. Calvin played pool with them after working in the bean fields. As he got better at pool, he eventually found a sucker. He hustled the guy, but it took a long time to beat him, with only the paltry win of about $40. He was complaining to Stitch about it and Stitch replied, "Hey man, you gotta realize, you gonna play pool or you gonna work. If you work, you not gonna play pool as good as you think." That's when Calvin said, "Forget the bean fields; let's get some money together and get out of here."

Even at his young age Calvin realized that while he had associations with people he had no real friends. His friends were really business associates, people who would be there to skim the cream, but never there to help him if and things turned sour. He learned at an early age not to rely on others to help.

However, getting out of a laborer's life wasn't quite as easy as it sounded. And making a life gambling wasn't always cake and ice cream either. Before Stitch and Calvin went on the road, Calvin had been following the seasons, moving from place to place to work in whatever crop fields were currently harvesting, whether it be in the Carolinas, Eastern seaboard, Maryland, or Virginia. In the 1950s the migrant worker was usually a Black Southerner or Puerto Rican, poor minorities who were generally the only populations at the time that would work as farm laborers.

One season Calvin jumped on one of the tramp trucks taking workers to harvest. He hadn't intended to work the fields, but rather to make extra money gambling. In the morning the boss knocked on the door and said, "Let's go, get up, we gotta go." "Go where?" thought Calvin, grudgingly. He soon found himself introduced to cucumbers with little spiny thorns. A day or two of that proved more than enough of cucumber picking. He caught a ride with someone going to Virginia.

The crops weren't ready there and Calvin was having a hard time making ends meet. Before long, at this young age, he became a wino, associating with winos, eating sardines and rice, getting drunk every day, telling stories, getting carried to his bunk when he could no longer walk. Life had not gone as Calvin had planned or dreamed.

Working and drinking his way from camp to camp down the Eastern seaboard, Calvin and an older fellow, James Williams, left walking one evening and ended up in a labor camp in Fort Pierce, Florida. James had heard somebody was hiring in one of the cane fields. They finally got jobs at the sugar mill, but Calvin admits that he wasn't a good laborer and never had a job he was happy with. They assigned him to hooking the trailers to the tractors, he recounts that the tractor drivers would back up as fast as Mario Andretti. In short order Calvin thought he was bound to lose his life, or at least his legs, with that job. So he asked for another and was given the job of chaining the tractors to the hoist that would lift the cane to the train that would take it into the mill. Yet again he found that there was little time to scramble away from being hoisted into the mill along with the cane and ground to fine dust. Once again he and James quit and this time they headed for Jacksonville, Florida.

They slept along the beaches, in and around Jacksonville, scraping by with the little they could get, pulling cardboard over themselves to keep warm when no wine or whiskey was there to do it for them. James also had a buddy in Jacksonville who let them sleep in his car for a few nights, but Calvin and James were awakened one morning in the doorway to a doctor's office in St. Augustine by a big-hearted lady who worked at a restaurant. James talked her into letting them work for a much-needed meal. After they did some dishwashing and cleaning, she fed them a huge meal and gave them about twelve dollars. He remembers her kindness, in spite of also remembering what a nightmare that whole trip was.

When he finally got his check from the Ft. Pierce mill, a paltry $40 or so, his shoes were so bad that they were almost non-existent. He cashed his check at a bar and a con man tried to swindle him out of that! Guess there's no honor among con men. A pair of shoes cost him $8 and the rest went for a ticket to Pahokee, Florida, a small town located directly on the shore of big Lake Okeechobee, the second largest fresh water lake in the United States, and his father's home. He remembers his daddy calling him "the prodigal son" as he made that walk up the street to return to his father.

He was welcomed home with a bar of lye soap and a bath, something Calvin had not had for quite some time. Each summer of his late teens, Calvin experienced the same type of escape, wandering from camp to camp trying to work his con and make a little money for himself and his family. Calvin's father had a favorite saying that an "old man's past is a young man's future." Calvin replied, in response to the man who he respected for his hard work in spite of his hard luck, "I've seen your past and I don't want it." This was never meant as disrespect for his father, only a prediction of Calvin's future.

Calvin's repertoire is full of stories about this period of Calvin's young life when he often was at the wrong place at the wrong time. Once while he, Otis and Stitch were cruising down the street in an Oldsmobile they had acquired a friend of theirs from Pahokee saw them and waved them down. "Friend, you all better get out of town!" he warned. He explained that the police were looking for two men, one of whom was a dead-ringer for Calvin. They left running scared and arrived in another small town about twelve miles away.

Otis kept the car when a contractor hired Stitch and Calvin to drive his truck to North Carolina to dig potatoes. Calvin, who didn't have a truck driver's license, was nonetheless driving the truck while Stitch dug potatoes, usually with no particular enthusiasm. Sometimes Calvin got down and helped just to make a little more headway. They weren't really nearly as interested in digging potatoes as in putting the foreman, Robert Jones, and his money in separate places.

Calvin was a wizard at cards and knew how to play "Georgia Skin." That game needs several people who bet their card remains in the deck longer than anyone else's. Of course, this meant that Calvin and Stitch used their chicanery again to shave and shape the cards so they could deal the cards to win. This was Calvin's idea of work, and he would spend as much time on card games, craps, and gambling as he could, sometimes all day long. They even loaded dice with lead so they knew how they would fall. They also trimmed dice, called shakes, which causes them to roll to the flat side so they knew what numbers would come up. These tricks are still a part of the gambling life in some arenas.

Then came pay day and they got about $700. Though it was not as much as they had hoped for, it was time to move on. They took part of their earnings and bought a panel wagon which would take them on up the eastern shore in search of other marks.

Calvin also recalls a time when he was about 17 years old and lived in the small town of Mount Dora with Otis and Stitch. Mount Dora, about two miles north of Orlando, has an elevation of 184 feet above sea level and qualifies it as a Mount in the mostly flat state of Florida. At one time citrus was the major industry in the area, with large shipments from Mount Dora. Calvin and the boys lived in a boarding house and did a little orange picking, but mostly hustling as they followed "the marks" up and down the Eastern seaboard.

His life as a flim flam man came to a screeching halt for a while in Pahokee where he and a partner had been playing the note game, a money-changing scam designed to confuse a money handling clerk into returning too much change. As Calvin tells it he was tired one evening when they stopped at a gas station while his partner went inside. Calvin warned him not to pull the scam on the attendant because they had already done it at that location too many times. The partner didn't listen, and the attendant discovered how he'd been cheated as the two were leaving. Unfortunately for them the boy wrote down the license plate and description of the car and reported it to the police. Not realizing what had transpired in the store, Calvin dropped off his partner and took the car, stopping at a restaurant. Police arrested him in the middle of his dinner of shrimp and fries, and also found and arrested his partner. Calvin spent sixty days in jail. "It was bad," remembers Calvin, "but it gave me time to evaluate my life."

He worked on a road crew chopping weeds, but when he returned to his cell an old alcoholic was there to preach to him. Calvin remembers well one particular homily of the old man..."Each man is going to be judged according to his deeds." His time in jail started him thinking about his hustler life and although his standards wouldn't allow him to out-and-out rob or do drugs, gambling and peddling were still a viable opportunity to make money. For the time being he lived by the hustler's code of "Do unto others as they would do unto you, only do it first."

After he was released from jail he continued to find any job he could catch, including garbage man and construction laborer. Once he got on the truck to work on a roofing job. When the boss looked at him and asked if he brought the necessary tools, which he hadn't, he said, "Yes." The boss asked why he didn't say, "Yes, sir." Calvin's reply was that his mommy and daddy taught him that "yes" was all that was necessary. He wasn't about to say, "Yes, sir, boss," to a white man. This was long before *Roots* but a sign that Calvin was never going to be downtrodden by the expectations for his race or situation.

In 1962 the United States placed a sugar embargo on Cuba because they expropriated properties of United States citizens and corporations. Since the U.S. was a major importer of Cuban sugar that then became unavailable, Florida farmers began planting much more sugar and stopped planting as much beans and corn. The American Blacks considered cutting cane demeaning so Haitians and other Caribbeans were hired for the task. Most of the cane cutters lived out of town so their ability to buy goods wasn't easy. Calvin, then nineteen, saw an opportunity, applied for and got his peddler's license. He started selling them whatever he could purchase wholesale in Miami, including clothes, jewelry, pots and pans— anything the immigrants might need.

When he got enough money together he decided he needed something to be remembered by, something to make other gamblers believe they were associating with the big time. He had noticed other hustlers with rubies and diamonds in their teeth so he had a dentist cement diamonds he purchased from a pawn shop in two upper adjacent incisor teeth. His CB handle was "Diamond Head." He sported these diamonds many years, until he felt they were actually detracting from what he was all about and didn't want to be considered a "clown act," or seen just as a Black man with diamonds in his teeth and had them removed. However, in 1976 during the US Open, Jack Nicklaus was being interviewed and commented, "I knew I was in trouble when I saw that guy with diamonds in his teeth."

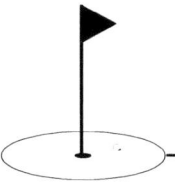

A New Course

Finally in 1966 when Calvin was twenty-three, some fellow hustlers talked him into taking a drive, one story has it they were going to a clambake, but Calvin doesn't remember clearly that detail. They also made a stop at the Genesee Valley Golf Club in Rochester, New York. This was the first time Calvin was exposed to the game of golf; he had previously thought it was only a game for old, rich white men. In fact, at one time on the more exclusive golf courses, not even Black caddies were allowed. Once that golf club was in his hands, he was hooked.

This was his way out of a life style that was probably leading to an early death from a knife or gun pulled by some guy who had been easily hustled. That wasn't an idea that was far-fetched as he already had personal experience of one such incident. Calvin recalls a time when he and a partner were shooting dice with a big mark–a fellow who could pay big, up to $6000. Of course, the game was heavily weighted to their side as Calvin had dice that had been altered. The game took a turn for the worse when one of the players accused them of cheating, which, of course, they were. The rest reads like a movie script! The fellow pulled a knife, but Calvin, fearing for his life, had a .32 caliber pistol in his belt and threatened to shoot the guy if he came at him. It must not have been a particularly good pistol as it misfired several times, but finally Calvin admits he shot the guy in the stomach. Still the guy kept coming at Calvin. Calvin's partner grabbed the gun and pulled the trigger, but again it misfired. Finally, Calvin's partner hit the guy in the head with the gun barrel, causing it to shoot. The guy dropped the knife and the two hustlers fled for their lives. It may sound more like a scene from a comedy, but it was real and Calvin knew that some day it was going to be deadly if he continued on the course his life had taken. As Calvin put it, "You had to be cool. If they saw you sweat they would know something was wrong. If they thought something was wrong, it could cost you your life, or your freedom."

Basketball superstar Michael Jordan once said, "Obstacles don't have to stop you. If you run into a wall, don't turn around and give up. Figure out how to climb it, go through it, or work around it." Calvin did just that. He realized that the old man's omen might come to pass ("you will be judged according to your deeds") if he didn't climb over the walls that surrounded his young, tough life. He had learned that he was ready to move on to respectability. Calvin's street life, however, ultimately was what made him the golfer he became.

During the time Calvin was growing up, golfers were generally restricted to playing certain courses. In 1926, long before Calvin was born, the United Golf Association was formed to promote the golf tournaments. A "Caucasian clause" in the Professional Golf Association's (PGA) rules excluded Black golfers from competing in the PGA tournaments until the early 1960s. At that time the NAACP, on behalf of Black golfers Bill Spiller and Ted Rhodes, took cases to the Supreme Court against golf courses that continued to promote segregation. In 1961 the PGA finally repealed its Caucasian-only clause. The fight for equality on the golf course was taken seriously by Joe Louis, Charlie Sifford, Ted Rhodes, Bill Spiller and Jackie Robinson. Upon their backs ride the likes of great Black golfers who have since competed in the PGA.

So finally in the 60's a Black golfer, Charlie Sifford, was allowed to play in and subsequently won both the Hartford Open and the Los Angeles Open. This was the same trailblazing Charlie Sifford who had been playing since before Calvin was born. The golf courses and even the PGA were still slow to promote Black golfers, and the introduction of the golf cart meant fewer opportunities for Blacks to learn the sport of golf as a caddy. Many Black players played the mini-tours as it was their only avenue to professional competition. Golf was still a white man's game and the restrictions against Blacks were manifold at the larger courses. Looking at photos of golfers and the gallery from the birth of golf to the beginning of Calvin's career will reveal very few Blacks. Not that Charlie or Calvin were the only Black trailblazers. John Shippen is recognized as the first golf pro and he played in the 1890s. And in 1899, Dr. George Grant, a Black dentist in Boston, invented and patented the first golf tee. Players before that used little mounds of sand to tee off from.

Many other Black players followed but until the 1960s they generally played the tournaments (often with purses as low as $100) sponsored by what was then known as the United States Colored Golf Association.

Calvin knew early on that he was a "quick study" of golf and that in order to compete at the pro level he had to be able to play at the better courses, to learn how to play the obstacles not apparent at the average public or country club golf courses. Many of these courses didn't see Black golfers, only cooks, janitors and caddies. Race and color were yet more obstacles he would have to strive to overcome, issues his perseverance and aptitude eventually minimized; at least as far as a golf career was concerned.

Calvin recalls, "One Sunday in 1968 I was rained out. As I went into the clubhouse, shaking off my rain suit, I looked up at the TV and saw a Black man tied for the lead with the best golfer in the world—Jack Nicklaus. That Black man was Lee Elder. They were playing in the American Golf Classic in Akron, Ohio. I thought 'There's a brother tied with the best golfer in the world!' That's when I thought if I give myself a few more years I could be out there on the tour, playing Lee Elder and the best golfers in the world. That was the beginning of my professional career."

Not many people, especially Black men over the age of 20 suddenly decide that they are going to be professional golfers. That Calvin did so under such difficult circumstances is a testament to his ability and determination.

"My golfing career really started in 1972 when I turned pro at the age of 29, an old man by today's standards. It was my era of mini-tours. In 1972, I won my first mini-tour, from Jim Salmon, a really nice guy. I shot 62 in Quail Hollow golf course north of Tampa in my first round. He shot 65 so I was 3 under." Going into the second round, Jim shot 65, and Calvin had a 3 shot lead which then tied them. Calvin said he was smiling at that point because he knew he couldn't lose. Calvin beat him at the playoff hole after having played golf for only six years. This was an amazing win for a golfer who could at that point still be considered a novice.

In 1975, at his first real tournament, Calvin states, "Lee Elder was very nice to me, he was my idol, and he told me that if there was anything he could do for me, maybe get me some exceptions, just ask. I thought no, if I can't earn it I don't deserve it." Although Calvin hadn't always earned his money the customary way, he refused to ask for favors or assume that others would help him out when things didn't quite go the way he had hoped. He remembers that back then he idolized Lee Elder as the first Black golfer to play in the Masters tournament. One day, he thought, he would be there, too, and do it on his own abilities, just as Elder had done.

"My grip was really bad and I had blisters on my hand from practicing. So I went to the drugstore and bought Dr. Scholl's foot pads and sewed them in my glove so I would still be able to practice. I was really a fanatic on practicing and within six months I broke 80 in my first golf tournament. That first real tournament was in Miami, the North & South Tournament, and was big with predominately Black players. Lee Elder and James Flack both played in that tournament." Most golf experts caution that when blisters occur it's from a bad grip and there are all kinds of remedies. Not one has mentioned Dr. Scholl's foot pads as a remedy. Calvin was inventing by necessity—the need to excel.

"I played many tournaments, many on country clubs, not municipal courses, and devoted my whole life to golf. Much like life, you have to be committed to what you do, to be better at it."

Calvin thought of golf as a science; thus once the basic concepts of the game were learned, it was simple. Then all that needed to be done was to practice those things that were learned. As he got better, he realized that golf is a game of angles, fractions, inches, a different angle at every hole. The next transition he made was body control and again it was a matter of practice. Calvin was always alone when he practiced, feeling that he didn't want to be around someone who was going to tell him what to do while he practiced. Robert Lynd, the Irish author, once said "It is difficult to remember how tragic the world is when playing golf." Perhaps there was a great deal of truth in that for Calvin.

Frequently in practice he would only hit short irons and wedges, and that's what helped him set up his timing, his rhythm, and increase his confidence because those clubs are usually easier to control. Then he would continue to increase up to a five-iron, which he considers the mid-range club.

As far as accuracy, timing, and rhythm were concerned he used the same philosophy as he did when he was hustling on the streets. It required the discipline to practice all day to be the best and to be good enough in his mind to have the confidence to go out and play. The difference was that instead of beating someone else at cards or craps, he was competing against himself and the golf course. Much the same way as he approached hustling on the streets, he had to find his own style and rhythm. He learned how to shift his weight from back foot to front foot during his swing, how to be accurate before learning the powerful drive. He found he couldn't copy those he learned from, but if he found a way that worked for him while learning the basics from them, he succeeded.

Practice is what helped him find his timing. If he didn't have the timing just right, he knew that the shot would be too fat, too thin, to the right or to the left. Calvin also found that getting the grip down was one of the hardest parts of the game to learn. He remarks that remembering how a grip should feel is something difficult, but practicing daily to grip the club is a must for a good game. "I learned later that the grip was one of the most important parts of the game. Through the hands is the only real connection to the ball." He also submits that eye and hand coordination is a matter of timing, knowing where your hands are supposed to be allows for everything else to follow. Those may be skills that he learned early in his hustling life.

"Charlie Sifford told me in Nashville when we were riding to a golf course one time that if he'd known how important the hands were in golf he would have been a much better player." Charlie, the trailblazer for many golfers, became Calvin's best friend on tour.

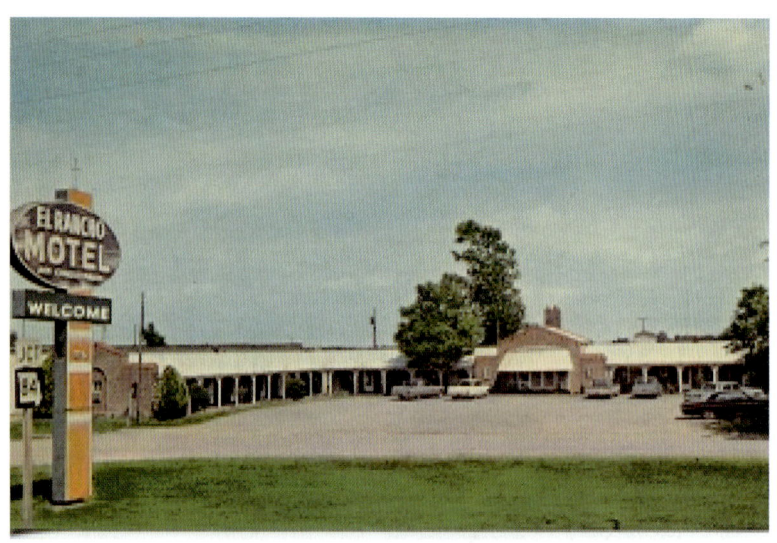

El Rancho Motel in Hayti, Missouri--better than Calvin's living quarters.

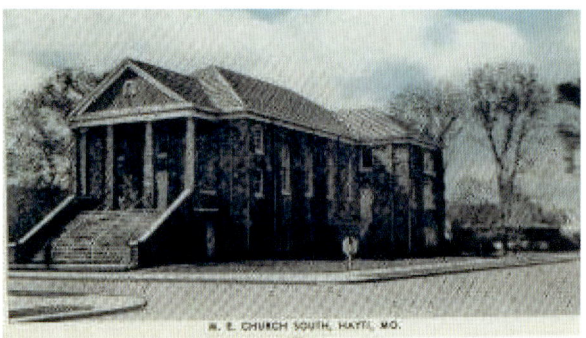

Old Church photo in Hayti, Missouri--probably not where he frequented.

For Peete's Sake 42

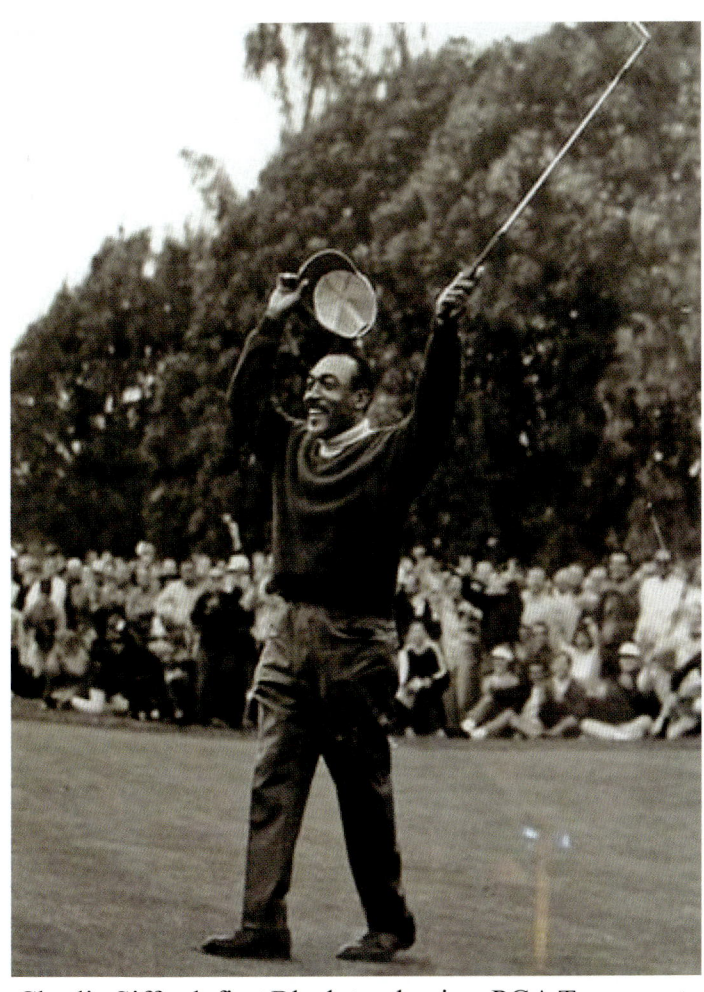

Charlie Sifford, first Black to play in a PGA Tour event, seen here without his signature cigar.

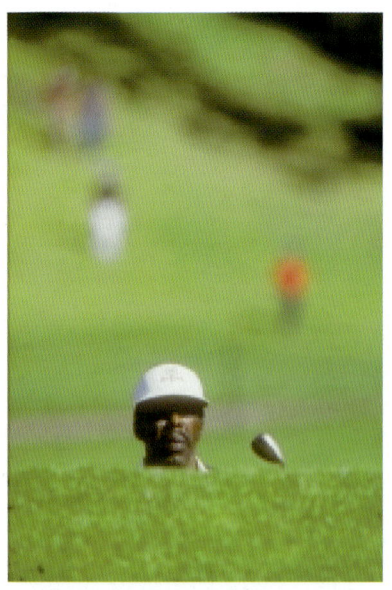

Calvin following the ball.

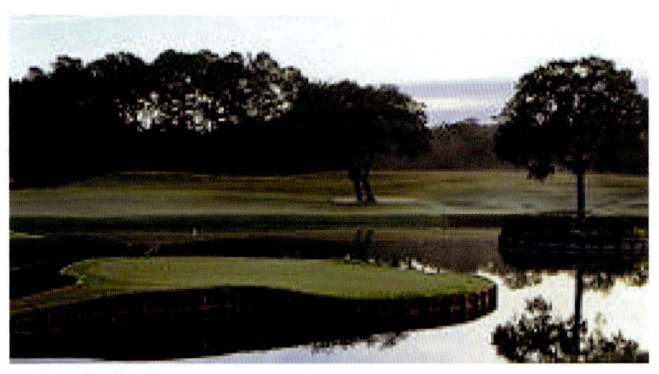

17th Hole on the Stadium Course at Sawgrass in Ponte Vedra, Florida.

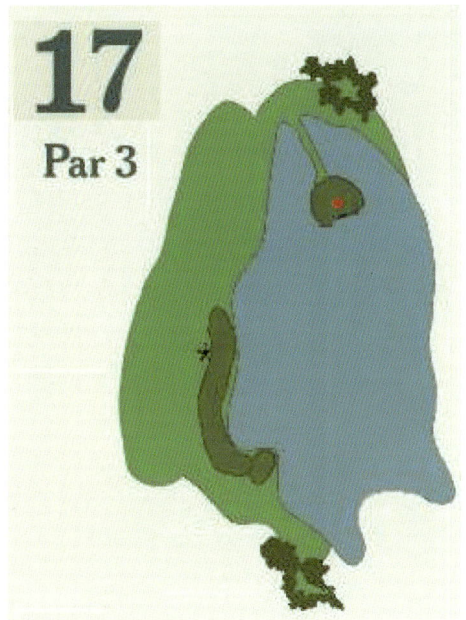

Map showing the 17th Hole at Sawgrass.

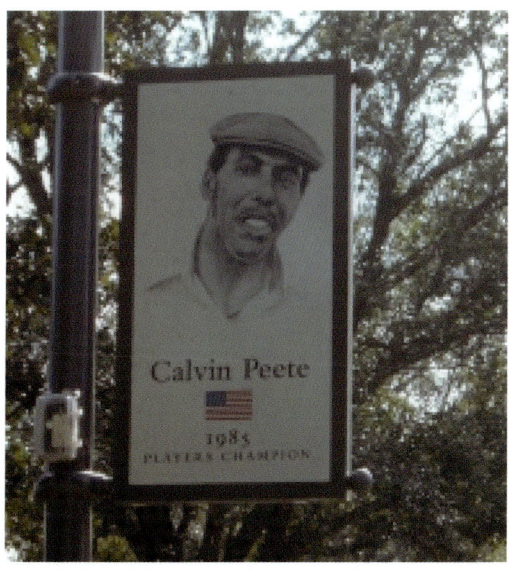

One of many permanent banner signs
along Champion's Boulevard at Sawgrass

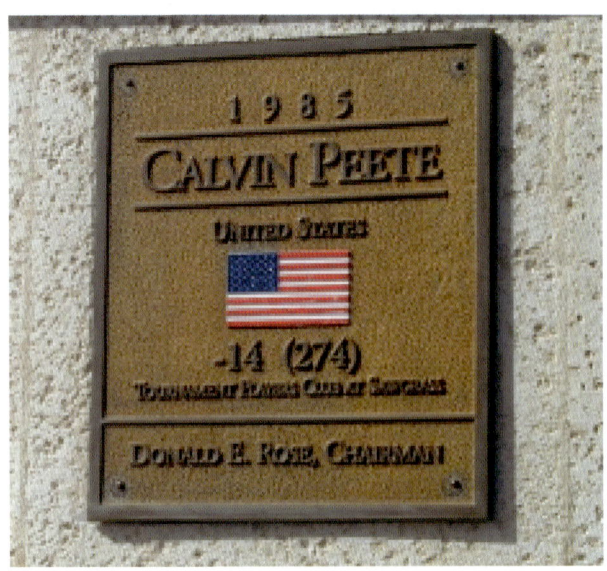

Placard on wall at Sawgrass Club House celebrating Calvin's 1985 win.

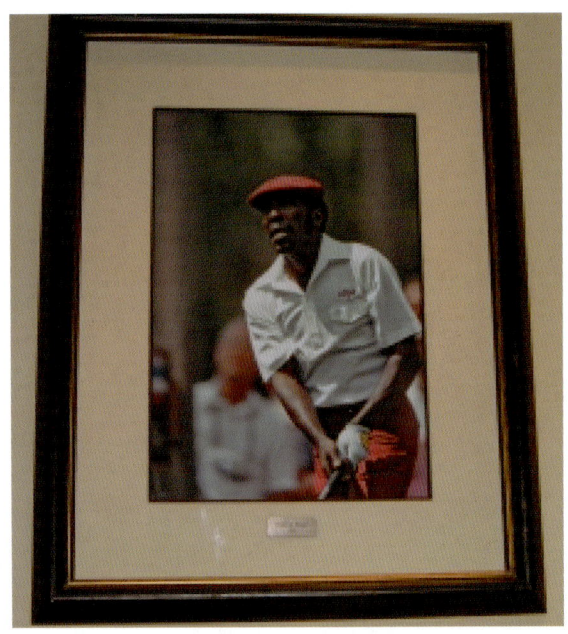

One of Calvin's photos in Sawgrass Club House.

For Peete's Sake 46

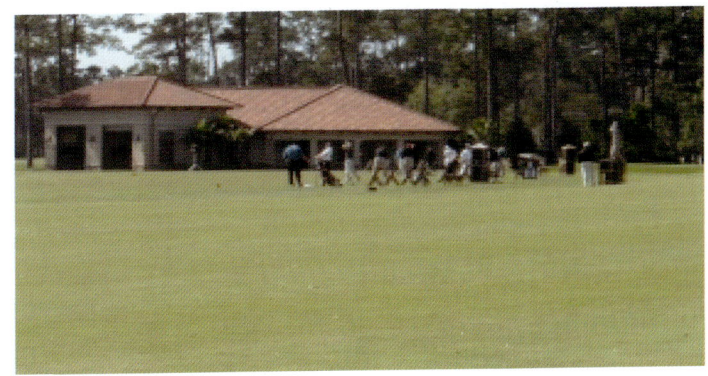
Sawgrass golfers on driving range.

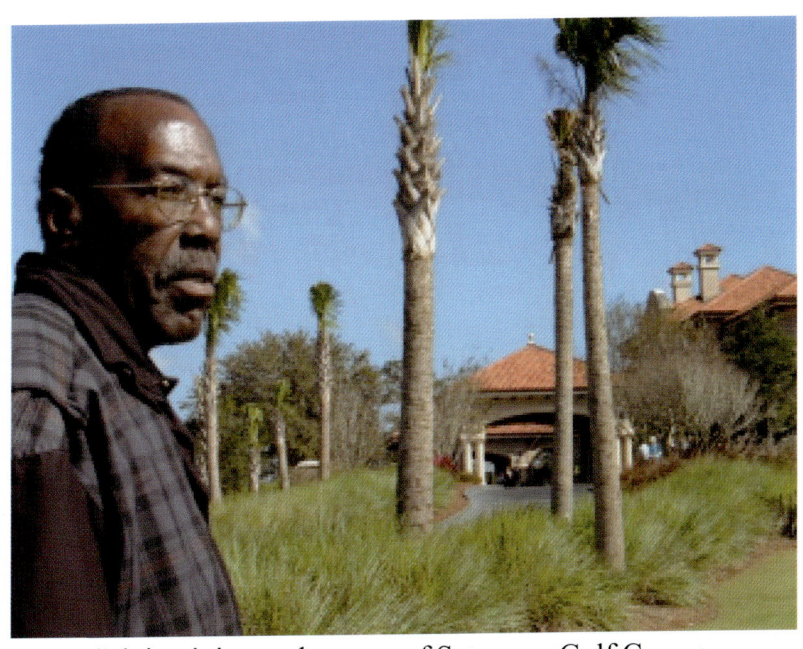
Calvin giving author tour of Sawgrass Golf Course.

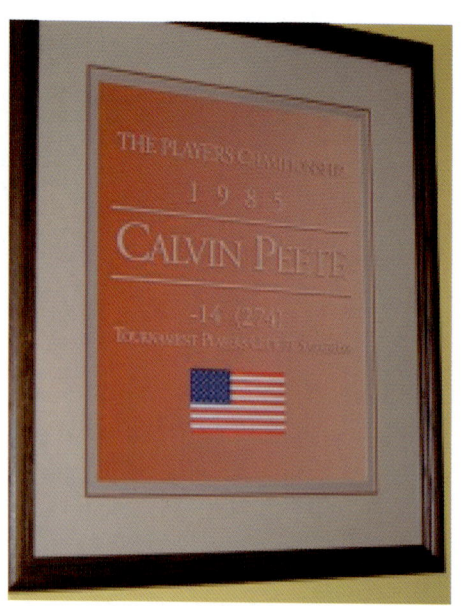

Framed Players Championship award
on Calvin's front room wall.

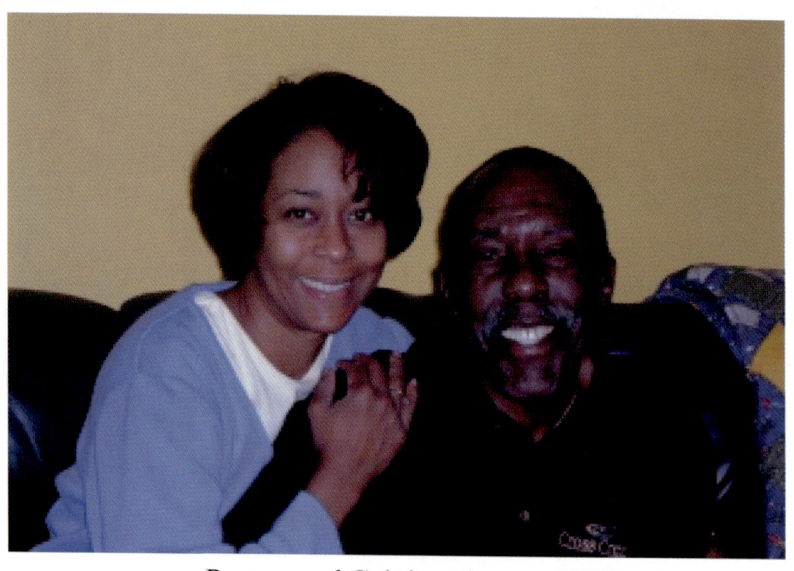

Pepper and Calvin at home--2008

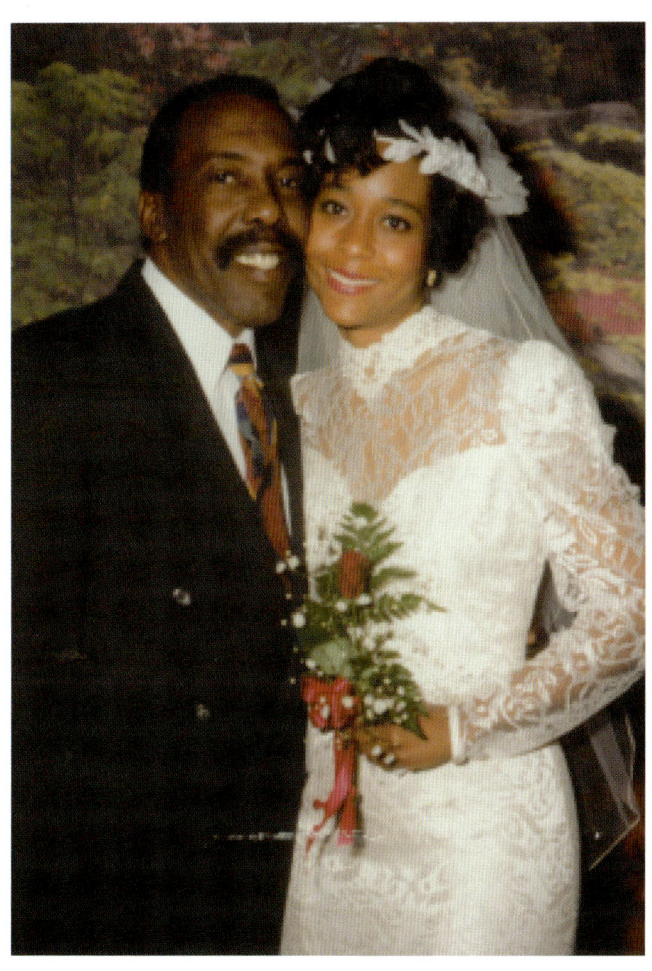

Calvin and his bride Pepper--1992

Nathaniel Starks, a Black PGA player in the 70s who Calvin holds in high esteem, told Calvin about a tournament in 1972 that was to be held in Dothan, Alabama, and urged him to go. It was a summer Calvin was playing very well, and Nate, as he was called, thought Calvin should be able to win. He did go, and it was the first time he ever felt nervous on the first tee and it showed when he hit the worst tee shot of his career. Then he talked himself up and got it together. It was such a long, tough golf course that there were only two golfers under par, one was Calvin at 2 under and the other was Tommy McGinnis at one under. Calvin won by one shot.

That gave him a lot of confidence. He knew he was not yet ready for the tour, but he qualified for regional, sectional and made it to the "school." For professional golfers the "school," or "Q-School" as it is often referred to, is not really a school at all. It is actually a group of qualifying tournaments that are used to qualify a fixed number of golfers to play in leading golf tours such as the U.S.-based PGA and LPGA tours. Getting through the school is extremely difficult and most professional golfers never succeed. The PGA's Tour Q-School has several stages of mini-tournaments. They are held in the fall in warm-weather locations in the U.S. A golfer who makes the cut in qualifying school wins membership of the tour for the following season, and holds a tour card that allows him to qualify on Monday to get in the tour tournament for the week. That means he can play in most of the tour's events without having to qualify as a player who has been on the previous year's money list. Players who are successful at Qualifying School can reach the elite level of competition very quickly. Explaining the Q-school is almost as difficult as graduating from it!

In order to go to the school, a player must pre-qualify. This means a letter must be submitted from three PGA Class A professional golfers attesting to the character of the applicant and the caliber of his golf game. These are submitted to the PGA Tour along with an application which includes a request for which section you'd like to play in. Then the PGA Tour sends the applicant a letter telling him which course he will go to pre-qualify for Qualifying School. Pre-qualifying also depends on how many spots are available. If the player qualifies where he is assigned, then it's on to regional qualifying, and once again, that depends on how many spots are available. All these are at the players' expense.

In 1972 and again in 1974 the school was in Napa, California. Calvin's first time through was a bust. His second try was during a cold, windy November, and Calvin didn't do too well, having less accuracy than he needed on the fairway and chipping it close to the hole. At that time he still hadn't realized angles and wind velocity played such a big part on the ball. He didn't qualify. By June 1975, he was continuing to have a good mini-tour career, and had acquired more experience.

During this phase of his life he met Christine. It was 1973 at a social function in Belle Glade, Florida, where he was introduced to her by a mutual friend. Calvin thought she was interesting, but he was focused on his career, and he already fathered three children, Calvin, Dennis, and Nicole and they were about all the responsibility he wanted, even though he seldom saw them. Christine already had a son, Ricky. But a year later when Christine became pregnant he married her and grew to love her and adopted Ricky who shares the Peete name, along with their new daughter, Kalvanetta.

Christine supported him while he worked on his golf skills. Through his golfing association with wealthy businessmen, he was able to acquire a large fifty-two unit apartment complex in Fort Lauderdale. That helped support his burgeoning family but unfortunately later burned to the ground. They were able to afford a lovely home in Fort Meyers after living their early married life in a trailer. Christine ran their business and tax shelter, Calvin Peete Enterprises, and worked out of a rented office. Eventually, Calvin's tax advisor said that was an unnecessary expense so they closed it.

Now once again in 1975 Calvin was ready to go to Qualifying School. Calvin had tried twice before making it to Qualifying School. There were seventy-five players who started in Calvin's school but only eleven qualified. This time Calvin made it, and never looked back.

The PGA Tour Qualifying Tournament is held in three stages at the end of each season. The top thirty place golfers and ties from the final stage (contested over 108 holes) gain membership and eligibility to play the subsequent calendar year on the PGA Tour. That year Calvin went to Qualifying School in Myrtle Beach, South Carolina, and the warm weather was perfect. Calvin usually doesn't like to play nor does he play his best in cold weather. On the way to Myrtle

Beach, with his wife, Chris, he hit a deer and wondered if it could possibly be a bad omen. It wasn't. They only gave out thirteen tour cards at that school, and Calvin was eighth in the class. After the class, a speaker came in and conducted a class on deportment on the course. Then the question was asked, "What makes you unique?" A young Native American replied, "I'm the only Indian." When Calvin was asked the question, his reply was, "I'm going to be the best golfer in the world," and, in fact he did become the best golfer in the world. That was the year Lee Elder became the first Black to play in the Masters.

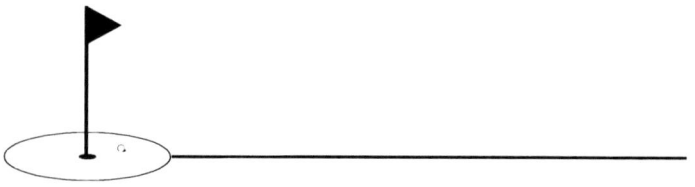

Time for the PGA Tour

Calvin's first tournament after qualifying for the PGA tour was in Milwaukee at the Greater Milwaukee Open July 1975. He was 6 under par after 26 holes, 2 shots back of the leader, and he missed the cut. A cut, or cut line, in a tournament is a score that represents the players that will play on and those that will be eliminated from the tournament. In this case the cut followed the second round of play. He took a 9 on the 18th hole, which was over par for the day. "It was a disaster." He shot long and short, hit bunkers, and did everything experience would have prevented. He looks on it as a blessing in disguise though, and four years later when once again in Milwaukee he proved how much better he had become at golf.

His next tournament in 1975 was in Moline, Illinois, at the Ed McMahon-Jaycees Quad City Open. According to Calvin, a gentleman, Lowell Biggs, followed him in the gallery and watched him play. Lee Elder was there and Lowell asked him about Calvin, but was never introduced to him. However, Calvin still wasn't at the top of his game and missed the cut again. The next week he missed the cut again in the Pleasant Valley Classic in Massachusetts, at one time a stop on the PGA tour circuit. Then there was a quick cross-country trip to a tournament in Massachusetts to qualify. Finally, he was in the play-off for the first spot. An official at that time, Pete Thissell, took him aside and encouraged Calvin by telling him that he was "going to be a good player."

He was now qualified but flat broke and in order to get back home he had to call his older brother, Ennis, for money. When he got home he called his father. His father relayed the message that Lowell Biggs, the gentleman who had previously followed and inquired about Calvin, had called and wanted to speak to Calvin when he got a chance. Calvin called Biggs who offered to sponsor him at $500 a week for six months, and it was settled as a gentleman's agreement.

Biggs sponsored Calvin for about six months before they even met, and that was a life-saver to Calvin during this time of struggle, both financially and professionally. Of course, Calvin's finances depended on his ability to win and that was still not always within his grip. Even during the Florida Winter Tour Lowell helped buy Calvin's children Christmas gifts and necessary items. Lowell Biggs was a businessman, farmer, and grocer, a man wealthy enough to support an upcoming golfer and insightful enough to realize that he was helping a future champion. After the six months was up they agreed contractually to a 50/50 split of the profits.

Lowell was an avid golfer who sponsored two other players–Mick Soli and Rusty Gurns. Lowell sponsored Calvin until 1984 when Calvin bought off his contract. Both men had made good money from Calvin's successes and ended their agreement on a friendly note. They still remain friends and even owned a golf course together for a while.

Calvin's mother died in 1976 while he was on tour. He had seen his mother only once since the time he had left home at age twelve. He saw her when at about nineteen he returned to Detroit to see his people. There is a notable sense of loss when he speaks of his mother, more significantly that her life's troubles kept her from seeing the strides he made in becoming a champion.

Calvin, married and with children, took his family with him when he did the summer tours. He had a van that they loaded up and they went on the road, usually filling at least a couple of motel or hotel rooms. It was a tough life, especially when he got to the real contender level. Now with a burgeoning family, the necessity of playing at a professional level, and always the undercurrent of race, it is a wonder that he didn't quit. But he didn't.

Calvin frequently talks about the sports press throughout his career and seems to have a poor opinion of many of its rank. He especially is disparaging of those who asked what he considers stupid questions such as, "How do you think you're going to do in the tournament?" Reporters, in his opinion, often seemed to have a poor knowledge of the golf game, having their expertise in other sports such as football, baseball, etc. However, Calvin remembered the etiquette rules he learned long ago at Q-school and handled their questions with style.

In 1979, Calvin again played the Greater Milwaukee Open which had a $30,000 prize, a great deal of money in those days. He knew he was playing well and worked hard not to let his confidence slide.

Golf is played as much in the mind as the body. He played steady, but the real contest was on the last day, when the tournament would be won or lost. With 19 under par and a total stroke count of 269 for 72 holes, five less than the closest contenders, he won in the last nine holes on Sunday, a tournament record at that time. A friend's telegram to him upon his win simply stated, "Stay hungry, Calvin."

He continued to play well in 1980 and 1981. Even though he didn't win a major tournament during those years, he earned over $100,000 each year. Again in 1982 he was back at the Greater Milwaukee Open. The large $200,000 purse had all the players smelling blood and Calvin led the tournament by one or two shots consistently and didn't make a mistake to crown his victory with his first place total of $45,000, his second tournament win that year. Now he was really being noticed and not for being a Black golfer, but for being an excellent golfer. Even though his childhood had been at times terrifying and miserable his time had finally come to be in command.

The year of 1982 continued to be a good year when Calvin played the Anheuser-Busch Classic in Williamsburg, Virginia. Another $30,000 purse would mean Calvin would have another significant year, but Hal Sutton was leading the field by six shots. Calvin, although playing a good, solid game, didn't expect to win. However, it all changed as Sutton failed to play consistently and Calvin won his second major tournament in a year. The gallery was amazed and didn't fail to notice that Calvin Peete was a player to be reckoned with.

Now really hitting his stride, he entered the 1982 B. C. Open, called the Broome County Open until 1971, at the En-Joie Golf Course, in Endicott, New York, just outside of Binghamton. With a purse identical to the others he had played for and won in 1982, almost $50,000, Calvin really hoped to play well. However, he was playing with two hot shots, Jerry Pate and Fuzzy Zoeller, who still didn't really give him much credence as an important player. Calvin's caddie told him that talk among Pate and Zoeller was that they each were playing for first and second. Calvin replied to his caddie, Bobby Morgan, "They don't know they are both playing for second." It set them on their heels when Calvin held out his second shot for eagle with a long iron and there was no looking back from there. He won with a tournament record at that time with 265 for 72 holes. That course record stood until 2005 when Jason Bohn shot a 264. Calvin also held the course 54-hole record that year of 196. Jerry Pate commented "You kicked both of our asses," and Calvin knew he had finally become a force to be reckoned with, a player who even the pro golfers would respect, something he so desperately wanted his whole life.

Calvin rounded out 1982 with the Pensacola Open and another $36,000 win. He'd been on the road quite a while and had decided to take three weeks off during which he didn't even practice, a rare thing for him. At the end of the three weeks he resumed practice and was surprised at how well he was still playing, hitting the ball solid and putting well on 18-20 footers, the area of the game that is so hard to master. So after Friday of the tournament he knew deep down that he wouldn't be beat. His adrenaline and excitement carried him through. Everyone was surprised by his win after such a long break. This may have been an ego-inflating win because Calvin knows he started 1983 a little "big-headed." But he continued from his PGA lead in 1982 through 1983 in driving accuracy, hitting more greens and fairways than anyone, and earning him the nickname, "Mr. Accuracy," a well-earned title that still stands today.

The year that he won four tournaments, 1982, came more than three years after he won in Milwaukee. "Winning that first time in Milwaukee may have been a fluke," comments Calvin. The following years he just tried to keep his exempt status from having to re-qualify to play in tournaments, to finish in the top sixty so he wouldn't have to qualify the next year. Knowing how hard it was when he originally qualified, he feared going through that grueling ordeal again. He paraphrases Jack Nicklaus here when he says, "That's the difference between a good player and a player that plays good." He admits that he played "good" at that time, but he wasn't a good player. Good players are always consistently near the top, really trying to win, and the player that plays "good" is simply trying to get a check. Then finally his attitude and his playing lived up to his potential, and he had become the player that he strived to be.

The proof of his skill and killer attitude in 1982 showed in his wins of The Greater Milwaukee Open for the second time, the Anheuser Busch Classic, the Pensacola Open, and the B.C. Open. He went on to win The Georgia Pacific Atlanta Golf Classic in 1983 but didn't win again until the Texas Open in 1984, even though he was still playing well enough to be making money.

    Calvin's most poignant memory of that Texas tournament was on Sunday morning when he was leading the tournament. Charlie Sifford was in town doing an exhibition on Monday and was staying at the same hotel as Calvin. Charlie invited Calvin to breakfast and as they sat chatting, Calvin mostly listened to Charlie's fascinating stories. Charlie talked about how he overcame many of the adversities of being a Black player, including the time when in 1952 he and boxing champion Joe Louis stepped to the first hole at the Phoenix Open and found human feces in the cup. Calvin had not experienced many of the discriminations and torment that Charlie Sifford had, but both of their lives had proven that adversity can make you strong. Finally, Charlie said, "Calvin, you know that you don't have anything to do with it right now, but I hope you win this @&#* tournament, because this is the only tournament that would not let Pete Brown and me in the gate when we were on tour together." Pete Brown was the first Black to win a PGA tour event, the 1964 Waco Turner Open. When Calvin won the Texas Open, an excitement of personal magnitude flooded him and he looked up and said, "Charlie, this is for you."

    Also in 1982, his managing company, IMG, booked him as a top player in Japan's Dunlop-Phoenix tournament, an annual November event on Japan's golf tour. This tournament attracts some of the leading international golfers, and Calvin was among those. He liked the greens there because they were small and tight and favored his title of Mr. Accuracy. His woman caddie said, "You ichibon." Calvin learned later that she said, "You're number one." He proved her right with his win when he played with Bobby Wadkins on their last round. He also played tournaments in England and France during his career.

Then in 1983, after winning four major tournaments, a number of smaller ones, and reaching the millionaire dollar winner mark, Calvin was chosen to play on the Ryder Cup team. For a poor Black boy who no one had expected to distinguish himself, this was an honor that exceeded even Calvin's expectations. However, in order to play in the Ryder's Cup a player must have a high school diploma or its equivalent. Calvin didn't. So, while on tour Christine tutored him and he studied hard and even managed eventually to get an honorary degree from his childhood home state college, Wayne University, by simply having a conversation with the Wayne State president. Imagine the honor bestowed on a man whose own grandmother had degraded him. Oh, if they could only have seen this!

The Ryder Cup is a golf team trophy challenge between the United States and Europe. It was named for Samuel Ryder, an English seed merchant and golf enthusiast who donated the trophy. Before 1983 it was between the U.S. and England, but the rules changed and the competition became keener. The top ten players in the PGA point system are selected. "It meant everything, representing my country and coming together with my previous rivals," states Calvin. Jack Nicklaus was the US Team captain and Tony Jacklin was the European Team captain for the match held at the Palm Beach Gardens, Florida, PGA National Golf Club. Jack did the pairings and Calvin was paired with Tom Kite for the morning foursomes, which Calvin thinks was a great selection.

The team competition between the golfers from both sides of the Atlantic is high, and that year after brutal intense golf the United States Team won the solid gold trophy by a narrow margin. Calvin's match on the last day was against Brian Waites, the European driving accuracy player for the year. Calvin says, "He was a formidable opponent, and the match was touch and go until the fourteenth hole. That's when I said to my caddie that I had to shake him off my ass. Then I birdie 14 and 15 to go two up with three to play, but then I came back a bogey 16 and we halved 17. We go into 18 and I am one up but I had to close him out. Five was a par 18 and he hit his third shot on the green. I did not think about his shot even though he was not close. I just thought about what I had to do right then. I hit the best shot of my career with a seven iron into a strong right-to-left wind. The shot ended up about six inches from the cup. The roar from the crowd was astounding."

Crowds were small and there were few stations broadcasting the tournament so the world would be slow to realize that Calvin was only the second Black golfer to play on the U.S. Ryder team. However, that same year Calvin also won the Golf Writers Ben Hogan Award which is presented annually to golfers who overcome physical handicaps or illness. Calvin's left arm was still not fully extendable due to his childhood fall, and some attribute his ability to be so consistent in his swing to this "disadvantage." To this day Calvin has the pin in his arm but it doesn't bother him.

The year 1984 continued to be a banner year when Calvin was presented with both the PGA's Vardon Trophy and the Byron Nelson Award for the player with the lowest scoring average per round (70.56). Calvin was at the top of his game as the first major golfer. He won more PGA tour events during the 1982-1985 years than any other golfer.

Lee Elder was his inspiration for the tour. He had seen Elder play with Jack Nicklaus one Sunday while watching television and was very impressed with him, playing "right down the middle." He said to himself, "In five or six more years I could be out there with Lee Elder." There were other players, too, that were inspirational to Calvin and he set goals based on the golfing of Lanny Watkins, Hale Erwin, Jack Nicklaus and Johnny Miller.

Interestingly, an anonymous blog quote says, "Calvin Peete is the guy who inspired me to start playing as a teenager back in 1984. He was one of my biggest childhood heroes." Many, many more young and old golfers, especially Black golfers, have found inspiration from the trials and successes of Calvin. However, Calvin felt that his ability to play golf was a gift from God, but perhaps a temporary gift. Eventually, he felt, that gift might have to be returned. The feeling was strong in 1984 and he looked to God for another two years, at least, before he sought what else he might do with his life.

Again in 1985, Calvin was high enough in points to be selected for the every-other-year Ryder Cup contest. This time it was held at The Belfry in Warwickshire, England, with Lee Trevino as U.S. and Tony Jacklin as European captains. This time "Tom

Kite and I probably were not the best combination, especially against the two from England." The U.S. Team lost badly and Europe won the tournament for the first time ever. Even though Calvin lost with his partner he won his singles match against Jose Rivero on Sunday. However, Calvin doesn't like bad weather and knows that affected his play in Britain and that's also "why I didn't play in the British Open."

In spite of the Ryder Cup loss and his decision not to play in the British Open, the year 1985 was another great year. In fact, it was probably the one Calvin is the most proud of and the one he probably is the most remembered for. He won the Tournament Players Championship (TPC) and the Phoenix Open.

In Phoenix he experienced problems with his right eye. He was wearing contact lenses at that time, and thought he might not have cleaned his hands well enough when he put his lenses in, even though he was meticulous about that detail. He was leading the tournament, but when he woke up Saturday morning he had a sharp pain in his right eye. It continued to get worse but he felt he couldn't withdraw—he was in the lead! His caddie at the time was "Golf Ball" Adolphus Hull. Calvin says he was probably one of the best caddies in the world as well as one of the first caddies on the professional tour. He told his caddie, "I can't see out of my right eye!" Golf Ball replied, "Just hang in there and do the best that you can." He struggled through in misery and ended the day at one over. There was an optometrist on the course who took Calvin to his office and checked his eye out but didn't find anything wrong. Calvin retired to his hotel and when he awoke the next morning his eye was clear with no pain. Calvin knew that was going to be his day! The win was his. Frequently, in any sport, how one plays the game depends less on the body than the mind.

The Stadium Course at the Tournament Players Club at Sawgrass in Ponte Vedra, Florida, usually referred to as the TPC at Sawgrass, was the course where the Tournament Players Championship was held in 1985. This tournament offers the highest prize fund of any tournament in golf and is sometimes called the Fifth Major although it does not have official major status. Calvin was not hitting the ball as well as he would have like to at the beginning of the week. On Wednesday of the tournament Calvin went to one of the trailers and changed his equipment, thinking that the problem he was having couldn't be with him (a trait that is common to professionals) but rather the club shafts that he had changed earlier. Once again he changed shafts, returning to his old ones.

After Saturday's round Calvin found himself tied for the lead. He went to bed early that night and woke up about 1:00 Sunday morning, unable to return to sleep. He decided to take a drive and while cruising down A1A he turned on his interior lights. Looking at himself in the rearview mirror, he said aloud, "This may be your only chance to win a tournament close to a major and when you are playing your best they can't beat you, and you are playing your best."

Back in his room on Sunday morning there was a knock at his door. His angel, his Daddy, arrived at his condo, having driven 300 miles and through two guard gates to be there. "I was so surprised to see him that my first question was, 'How did you find me?" His father answered, "No matter where you are, boy, I'll find you." Calvin loved that and knew that he could not be beat that day. It was the first tournament his father had ever seen him play in, and he walked the whole 18 holes.

He was tied for the lead going into the last round. His confidence was high, his adrenaline was high, and a streets attitude of "no fear" carried him through. Calvin can recall exactly how he played each hole—bogey, birdie, or par—which club he used, his stance and swing, and the excitement when the ball soared to exactly where he wanted it. "I started the first hole birdie, the second hole birdie, and quickly took a two-shot lead and never looked back. It was up to a four shot lead by the time we made the turn." But D.A. Weibring shaved that four shot lead down to two by the time they got to the seventeen.

Stadium Course's Par 3, 137-yard hole #17, is instantly recognizable to golf fans worldwide as "the Island Green" because it is almost completely surrounded by water. It is what has become the TPC Sawgrass signature hole, the hole that holds the audience spellbound, and the most famous par 3 in golf. Calvin's knees, "felt like mush, and it was the first time in my whole career that I felt fear." He reminded himself that this shot was what he'd hit all those balls for, what he had spent all that time practicing for.

It was here that Calvin shot one of the best shots of his career under the circumstances—an eight iron to within five feet of the pin for a 3-shot lead, and the crowd exploded. It was the shot heard all over the world. He went on to make the put and take a three shot lead going into the eighteenth hole. With water all down the left side of the eighteenth hole his driving accuracy hit a great drive down the right side of the fairway. He hit a six iron into the green that just trickled off the back edge about a foot with the pin in the back. It was an easy two-putt to win the Championship. His final round of 66 cinched the 1985 Tournament Players Championship. At age forty-one he had birdied the 17th hole and with 14-under 274 set a new TPC Sawgrass tournament record and became the oldest player to take the title. So ten years after the Q-school when he said he could be the best golfer in the world, he proved it. At this point he was the best golfer in the world. Calvin remembers, "Hale Irwin congratulated me on my victory and said that it was the best round of golf that he had ever witnessed."

Only three other players in their forties have won this tournament. Golf, however, doesn't always rely on age or power, but precision, Calvin's specialty. Calvin's name is on the list of winners for this tournament along with other great golfers such as Jack Nicklaus, Lee Trevino, Raymond Floyd, David Duvall, Phil Mickelson, and Hal Sutton. The list, of course, includes many other great golfers, but few, if any, have struggled so hard to accomplish so much with so many hurdles to jump. Calvin proved undeniably that he is a champion among champions. The world looks now to a new era of golf. The game has changed enormously from the time of Charlie Sifford, Jack Nicklaus, Arnold Palmer, Lee Trevino, and Gary Player. Those were Calvin's heroes and their names have become synonymous with great golf. But the name Calvin Peete should always be on the list of great golfers, and a hero to all who aspire to be better in life.

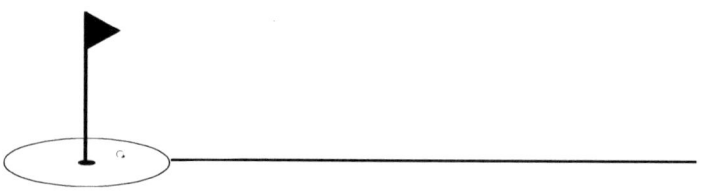

1986
Tournament of Champions

"I don't know what happened. Tapping and missing, tapping and missing. I wasn't myself." Eventually, at the 1985 Tournament of Champions, even though he was playing in a twosome with Curtis Strange, he would not withdraw. Though he could not accurately record the score on that hole, he did finish the round. However, after finishing the round he called the officials and disqualified himself. One of Calvin's strongest features became his downfall—his perfectionism. If he didn't play well he didn't want to play at all. He was guaranteed $4000, but it was withheld as a fine, a penalty for withdrawing, considered conduct unbecoming a professional, which Calvin agrees with.

The next year, 1986, at the La Costa Club in Carlsbad, California, he returned with a vengeance. He had been practicing all winter, working hard on his game, not putting his clubs in the garage like he usually would after the tour break. With 21 under, a course record, Calvin had no problem redeeming himself at the MONY Tournament of Champions. His six shots over his closest rival set a new tournament victory record, the lowest total score of his career. As he made his trophy acceptance speech he apologized to the people of Carlsbad for his previous year's conduct.

In 1986 he was in New Orleans at the USF&G Classic (now called the Zurich Classic). Calvin, who was then forty-three-years old, had a disc problem in his back, and was playing against much younger players. But the year had been good to him and he was driving, playing, and hitting good iron shots, not worrying about making mistakes. He had a two-shot lead going into the final round. Unfortunately the round was rained out on Saturday, so the players, young and old, had to play thirty-six holes on Sunday. The press questioned him on whether he could hold up to thirty-six holes against the younger players. "You ask me after the last hole and we'll see how they hold up," replied Calvin. Calvin knew that he was playing well so thirty-six holes was something he could do easily and it wouldn't bother him. He won that tournament easily with 19 under and a purse of $54,000.

He was in the money again in 1986 from the MONY Tournament of Champions in California where he won $90,000 by golfing 21 under par for the tournament record, which still stands. At 267 he won by 7 strokes under Mark O'Meara and even greater margins against Hal Sutton, Jim Thorpe, and Fuzzy Zoeller. He still feels that was his best tournament ever and remembers he just felt good about the course and that the gallery saw him always in the lead. He finished twelfth on the PGA earnings list that year.

Eventually the years of living on the road and the challenges of marriage caught up to him. He asked

Christine for a divorce in 1987. According to Calvin, her spending had gotten out of hand. The four years from 1982 to 1986 were spent in marital turmoil, with constant disagreements about the large amounts of money she was spending. His accountant cautioned him that they couldn't keep up the life style she was creating. Calvin gave her the house and agreed to pay for the children's college in a civil divorce. There were no arguments with the settlement. Christine was comfortable with the decision to be Christine Peete, not always an appendage to Calvin Peete. Their only child from the marriage, Kalvanetta, was about twelve at the time. He still sees and talks to all of his children and Christine, who has never remarried, is included in some family get-togethers.

When Calvin told his father that he and Christine were divorcing, he added, "I'm leaving Chris, but not my kids like you did." His father was crestfallen but Calvin assured him that he wasn't angry but simply remembered how miserable his childhood had been when his father left. He eventually died of prostate cancer in a rest home at the age of eighty-four. Ceatris, his stepmother, died of an aneurism and her children have never maintained a relationship with Calvin and his other siblings from his father's first marriage.

Calvin had two more years of great success, but in 1987 the new journey was beginning. His desire to play professional golf had dwindled, although he had contracts and a family to care for. He needed the checks from Coca Cola and his other sponsors. He still was having trouble with his eyesight, and an optometrist sent him to a doctor in Hartford. She gave him an association test and told him that his "eyes and brain weren't communicating." She suggested that he use colored balls, but he didn't feel that helped. He found he had to use reverse psychology on himself, telling himself to play left when he knew he should play right, doing the opposite of what he knew should be done. He knew something still wasn't right but didn't know what it was.

While playing in the Phoenix Open in 1987 Calvin, now single, attended a social at the golf club. There he was introduced to a young woman, an amateur golfer, by her father, an avid golfer who had won many private tournaments. Her name was Elaine Pepper Bolden and as they talked they found they had a lot in common, including their desire to be elsewhere at that moment. Barry Bonds, the man who later would be a baseball superstar, was at that gathering and was impressed enough to get Calvin's autograph, but Calvin was even more impressed with young Pepper. She in turn was taken with Calvin, and since she had been playing golf from an early age, her father had told her how much he admired Calvin's golf record. They danced their first dance to Billy Ocean's, "Caribbean Queen." They were soon inseparable. Friends had asked him repeatedly through the years if they were married. Finally, on a plane flying back from a tournament in Mexico City, Calvin proposed, knowing he could never, ever do any better. Pepper said, "Yes" and they were married in 1992 in "The Little White Chapel" in Las Vegas with golfing friend Larry Marks and his wife, Barbara, as witnesses.

Calvin won twelve events in the United States and one in Japan. In all, he played twenty seven or twenty eight tournaments a year, including four or five in Japan. But a steady diet of tournaments was not to his benefit or liking, and his position and earnings plummeted in the years following 1986. He finished in only six of twenty-five tournaments by 1990, two of eleven in 1991 and none of five that he entered in 1992. In fact, in 1992 he was forced to drop out of the 1992 Player's Championship because of the pain from of a later-diagnosed torn rotator cuff.

His favorite courses include all those he won on– -12 total but because he won two tournaments twice he really only has 10 favorites. The Harbortown course at Hilton Head remains the one he enjoyed the most, even though he had some not-so-good finishes. His best finish was fourth, but it was a course that he felt that he could win on. It was a prime example that a golf course didn't have to be seventy-five hundred yards to be considered a good golf course. He states that the best golf course in his opinion is the one where the best shot-maker wins, not one that demands brute force, which seems to be the current standard.

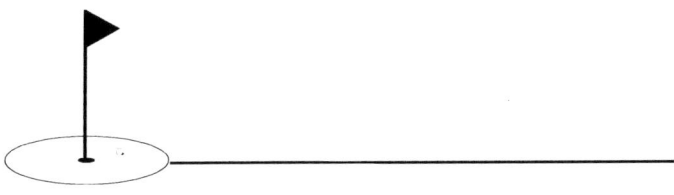

Yet Another Setback

Calvin struggled with his playing for several years before finally being diagnosed with Tourette syndrome (TS) in 1999. Tourette syndrome is a neurological disorder, according to the National Institutes of Health, characterized by repetitive, stereotyped, involuntary muscle group movements and vocal outbursts called tics. The disorder is named for Dr. Georges Gilles de la Tourette, the pioneering French neurologist who in 1885 first described the condition in an eighty-six-year-old French noblewoman.

The early symptoms of TS are almost always noticed first in childhood, with the average onset between the ages of seven and ten years. TS occurs in people from all ethnic groups; males are affected about three to four times more often than females. It is estimated that 200,000 Americans have the most severe form of TS, and as many as one in a hundred exhibit milder and less complex symptoms such as chronic motor or vocal tics or transient tics during childhood. Although TS can be a chronic condition with symptoms lasting a lifetime, most people with the condition experience their worst symptoms in their early teens, with improvement occurring in the late teens and continuing into adulthood.

In Calvin's case his symptoms were neither recognized nor treated, probably because of his environment of too many children growing up in poverty and neglect. Tics are the most recognizable physical manifestation of the condition, such as eye blinking, shoulder shrugging, facial grimaces. There are numerous other symptoms that can include head banging, eye poking and lip biting which are all classified as motor tics. In addition, obsessive-compulsive disorder, attention-deficit-hyperactivity disorder, learning disabilities, mood changes which cause behavioral problems are all commonly associated conditions in Tourette syndrome. However, the general public usually associates Tourette syndrome with the more aggressive vocal exclamation of obscene words or socially inappropriate and derogatory remarks (coprolalia). This thinking is a result of much disinformation generated by the movie, television and video industry sensationalizing the rarer symptoms of Tourette syndrome.

Calvin remembers certain unusual things he did as a child, such as moving his jaw up and down. His mother constantly reprimanded him and demanded he stop doing that and eventually it went away, but returned later in a different manifestation–moving his jaw side to side. His inability to pay attention to school, even his falling from the tree could have been associated with TS. No one paid much attention to it, but upon his Tourette syndrome diagnosis, the realization that Calvin had won many PGA tournaments in spite of this condition astounded his doctors. Calvin also wonders how he had such success when he looks back over the symptoms he had. Only approximately ten percent of adults have a progressive or disabling course that lasts into adulthood. Calvin is one of those ten percent.

Before that diagnosis and at the age of forty-three he knew he wasn't up to his previous abilities or even his competitive desire to play great golf. However, life goes on, contracts demand, and families need to be taken care of. And Calvin's family was expanding. Pepper and Calvin had their first child Elaine Aisha, whom they call Aisha, November 30, 1993. She started traveling on the tour with her parents when she was only twelve weeks old. Golfers always talked to Pepper and admired the baby as she pushed the stroller around the courses Calvin played.

On Aug. 19, 1996, Aisha was followed by a sister Ireanna Aleya, called Aleya. Pepper would occasionally take both girls to watch Calvin play, but toddlers were often at bit more than she could handle at a golf course. This was also the year Calvin made his first hole-in-one at the Silverado Country Club in Napa, California. He signed the ball and gave it to his baby daughter, Aleya, who still shows it with pride.

They all now live in Ponte Vedra, Florida, near the Sawgrass Golf Course where Calvin is a lifetime member. The girls are beautiful young women actively involved in school, dance and, of course, golf. The girls are each other's best friends and they hope, as their parents do, that they will get golf scholarships for college.

At the age of fifty Calvin began playing in the Senior, or Champions Tour. But this was the stage of his life when his tics were the most prominent. Young people are usually told that their symptoms of TS will lessen as they grow older, but with Calvin that was not the case. Involuntary muscle spasms worried him, and his use of verbal obscenities on a public golf course left him feeling that he should be in a mental institution, not playing golf. He was talking back to himself, aloud and as if to his demon, saying things like, "Why don't you leave me alone?" Pepper, his wife, supported him through those times, and encouraged him to seek help. However, the medication he was given on diagnosis did not seem to alleviate his problems.

In an effort to control his movements he tried both meds and occasionally alcohol when he wasn't golfing, but they only helped for a short time before requiring more and more. This was a time when Calvin acquired the reputation in the golf world of having a drinking problem; most people didn't know that it really was a time of uncontrollable tics. He feels his biggest help was God and prayer. Minister Isador Edward, a minister from Fort Worth, Texas, counseled and mentored Calvin. His problems diminished as his church attendance increased. Calvin knows that he is one of the lucky ones with Tourette syndrome, as his symptoms are not nearly as severe as many who have it.

In 1997 Dr. Lin at the Mayo Clinic examined Calvin and told him that his Tourette syndrome was not chronic, or in other words, Calvin's tic behavior is not always present. In fact, on many days, one would not know that Calvin has a motor or vocal tic. He tried the drugs Dr. Lin prescribed but didn't like the side effects, and told him that he no longer wanted to be on them. Current medications sometimes cause more trouble than the tics and there is no treatment that will cure TS. He now doesn't take any drugs, not even pain killers for his neck and shoulder pain, which is a complication or comorbid disorder as a result of the tics.

By the late 90s his disability affected his game so severely that his level of play hit some extreme lows. He was no longer among the champion golfers and he knew it. He says "I knew I just couldn't do it any more. I had to quit torturing myself and find out how to deal with this." The stress of worrying about his game and competing caused the symptoms of his disorder to intensify. So in 2001 he made the decision to retire at the age of fifty-eight. It was a hard decision to make, but he knew it was the right one.

Shortly after Calvin retired, the PGA went into partnership with a golf school and it founded the PGA Tour/PGA Tour Golf Academy at the World Village in St. Augustine, Florida. Calvin taught there for a couple of years but his Tourette's syndrome caused his attention span to be so short he didn't feel he was giving the quality guidance to his students that he should.

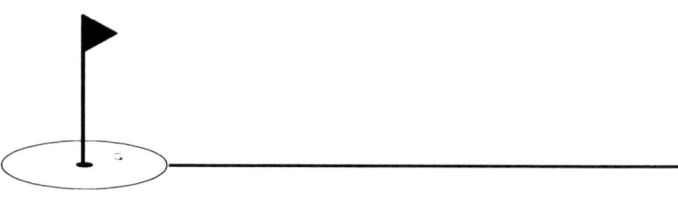

A New View

The 9/11 attack on the World Trade Center and the Pentagon caused the world to take a time to reflect. Golf was not an exception. Events such as the Tampa Bay Classic and Senior PGA Tour and the LPGA Tour were called off. The Ryder Cup was postponed for a year. When events were scheduled security was heightened. Calvin's attention turned to Pepper and his family, as it did for many Americans. It was time to show how much he appreciated their support through the years.

Looking back, he saw how his family was often neglected as far as having his attention. He was constantly gone, even though that provided well for them, and his children benefited by receiving good educations and rewarding jobs, they did not experience a close relationship with their father.

Calvin is proud of all of his children and their accomplishments. Indeed, his five older children lead successful lives and never experienced the kind of childhood that Calvin did. His oldest son, Calvin Peete Junior, born in 1968, attended Northwestern University and is a real estate broker in Baltimore, Maryland. Dennis, named after Calvin's father and born in 1969, is a mechanical engineer. Ricky, Christine's son born in 1969 and Calvin's adopted son, went to the University of Virginia and is an IT technician. Nicole, born in 1973, graduated from Alabama State University and is a teacher continuing her education towards a Ph.D. Kalvanetta graduated from Florida State University, received her law degree, and is currently studying for the Bar.

Calvin didn't want the same life for his "second family." He wanted truly to be there for them, thus influencing his decision to retire. He feels that retirement has been an important gift to him, bringing him closer to God and family. Things that he hadn't considered when in the streets, or on tour, now have become paramount. He and Pepper are settled in a charming gated community near the Tournament Players Club where they have lived for more than sixteen years.

Pepper works as the Executive Director for the First Tee of Jacksonville, a non-profit foundation dedicated to life enrichment through golf for young people eight through eighteen. Coincidentally, Joe Louis Barrow, the son of the famous prizefighter and golfer, Joe Louis, who Calvin met as a child, is the National First Tee CEO. Pepper also met Joe Louis when she was seven, like little Calvin. After she met his son, Louis, at First Tee, she told him how his father had influenced Calvin.

Pepper started at First Tee as an instructor and has gradually worked her way to the top and is now heavily involved in fund raising. Calvin is as proud of Pepper as she has been of him, and remarks, "I never wanted to overshadow my wife. She's the celebrity now."

Of course, Calvin's modesty belies the fact that he could stand as inspiration and role model for any young golfer today. Often a person with an underprivileged or handicapped beginning will make superhuman efforts to overcome it. The Greek orator Demosthenes had such severe speech problems he could hardly be understood. So he shut himself up in his study or escaped by himself to the beach, put pebbles in his mouth and practiced where no one could see or hear him. Ultimately he became one of the most celebrated orators in a nation of orators. Much like Demosthenes Calvin's life is a reflection of what utmost capabilities can be demonstrated in spite of extreme difficulties and limitations.

Now he spends much of his time in meditation and prayer. He's often home when his children return from school. He is in contact with his grown children and nine grandchildren, and his remaining brothers and sisters. These are ways he feels will help him get better, become wiser. He philosophizes about his illness: "In a biblical sense, if this (Tourette syndrome) had happened when I was a child, I wouldn't be here. God turned it around."

Calvin has felt privileged to meet many famous people, not all of them in the golf profession. He cites names like Sidney Poitier, Oprah Winfrey, Richard Roundtree, Clifton Davis, Mohammed Ali, Robert Wagner, Sean Connery, Kevin Costner, Dr. J, Magic Johnson, and Billy Dee Williams to list a few of those he's met, and, of course, Joe Louis.

Historically, all of the Blacks (Calvin being an exception) who played professional golf came up through the caddie ranks. Now caddies are an endangered species. These days a golfer usually needs to compete through the college ranks, be drafted for a college team, to get a chance to be a pro.

Technology also has changed the game. Club material allows the ball to be hit further. However, Calvin feels courses should be made tighter, rather than longer, and that would weed out the power golfers from the better, more accurate golfers. Expertise and precision should be the key elements when a player strives to be a champion. He added, "Ability is the most important attribute for a golfer. With my precision I lifted the bar and made other players get better." Calvin's record of winning 11 PGA Tour events and leading the tour in driving accuracy for ten consecutive years should be proof of his ability. But he also led the tour statistics for greens in regulation three times, was a U.S. Ryder Cup team member twice and earned more than $3 million on the PGA and Champions tours. Certainly he has earned the respect and admiration of other Black golfers who have followed in his very large footsteps.

Calvin is called upon to be a motivational speaker for corporate events and at exhibition golf events. His theme is, "When I realized I had the potential to be the best, I was motivated to become the best." He recounts that in golf one needs to motivate oneself. He informs his audiences that he was not intimidated by the gallery, in fact, he would feed off of it. But it was important to him that he would not embarrass himself in front of all those people. He reminds people that nobody expected Blacks to reach the heights they have in sports least of all golf and tennis.

Few expected Calvin's golf career to last more than a year or two. In fact, Calvin has said, "By all statistics I should be someone breaking into your home." He also reminds his listeners that golf is a lonely sport, requiring practice alone in all kinds of weather. Calvin had about fifty notebooks on practice tips, evidence of his dedication to the sport. Unfortunately they were inadvertently thrown away when they moved to Ponte Vedra. Such a huge collection of guidance would be invaluable to anyone interested in the finer points of golf.

Calvin can still be contacted for speaking engagements and likes family-type groups, especially if there are young people he can motivate. He frequently gives 30-minute seminars of golf tips at outings. He never heard anyone do that when he was young and would like to be that voice now, imparting what he has learned the hard way about what can be done, achieved, accomplished.

He speaks from experience when telling people that they "don't have to have a Ph.D. to be successful. We can all function with some kind of defect." Certainly he has proven throughout his lifetime of adversities that no matter what color your skin, no matter what hardships one faces, no matter how insurmountable the odds seem to be, a winner mentality can overcome all.

Defect, weakness, imperfection, disadvantage all can be applied to Calvin Peete. Ambitious, able, indefatigable, successful can also be used to describe him. Whatever words you use, the ones used most often are champion, winner.

Statistics

Born 7/18/1943 in Detroit, Michigan

Residence in Ponte Vedra, Florida

Turned Pro in 1975

Height is 5'10"

Family: Father: Dennis Peete

Mother: Irene Bridgeford Peete

Siblings: Iris, Aaron, Rachel, Dennis, Ennis, Irene, Margaret

Children: Calvin, Jr., Dennis, Nicole, Kalvanetta, Ricky (Adopted), Aisha, Aleya

PGA Golf History

Most successful Black (African American) player on the PGA tour until recently.

1979:   Greater Milwaukee Open

1982:   Greater Milwaukee Open; Anheuser-Busch Classic; B.C. Open; Pensacola Open

1983:   Georgia Pacific Atlanta Golf Classic; ` Anheuser-Busch Classic

1984:   Texas Open

1985   Phoenix Open; Tournament Players Championship

1986:   MONY Tournament of Champions, USF&G Classic

Awards

"Most Improved Player" Award, Golf Digest; led PGA in driving accuracy and greens in regulation strokes, 1982 and 1983; member of U.S. Ryder Cup team, 1983 & 1985; honorary degree, Wayne State University, 1983; Ben Hogan Award, Golf Writers Association, 1983; Jackie Robinson Award, 1983; two-time winner of Vardon Trophy (lowest scoring average per round); named to Golf magazine's All-American team: Black Achievement Award, Ebony.

About the Author

Dolly Ness was born in Butte, Montana, and graduated from the University of Montana with a degree in English Education. She has worn many hats: teacher, business owner and manager, government worker, and freelance writer. She is the author of various magazine articles but this is her first book. She lives in Newport, Oregon, with her husband, Troy, and Cavalier King Charles dog, Duffy.

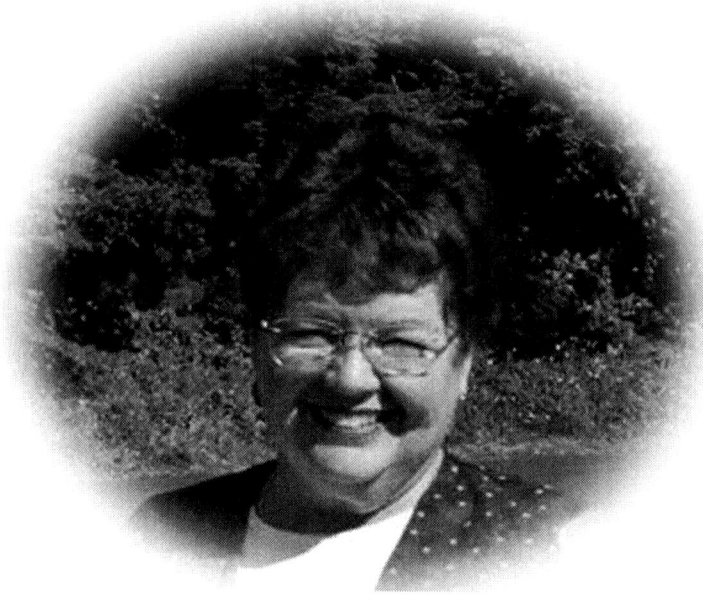

Dolly Ness